National Health

Editor: Tracy Biram

Volume 392

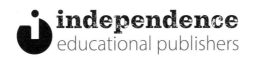

independence
educational publishers

First published by Independence Educational Publishers

The Studio, High Green

Great Shelford

Cambridge CB22 5EG

England

ISBN-13: 978 1 86168 850 7

Printed in Great Britain

Zenith Print Group

Contents

Introduction

National Health is Volume 392 in the **issues** series. The aim of the series is to offer current, diverse information about important issues in our world, from a UK perspective.

ABOUT NATIONAL HEALTH

The coronavirus pandemic has presented the biggest threat to our health as a nation this century. The challenges faced by the already struggling NHS have been unprecedented. This book looks at the impact of COVID-19, budget cuts and staffing shortages, as well as exploring the common health issues and illnesses that continue to ail us across the UK.

OUR SOURCES

Titles in the **issues** series are designed to function as educational resource books, providing a balanced overview of a specific subject.

The information in our books is comprised of facts, articles and opinions from many different sources, including:

- Newspaper reports and opinion pieces
- Website factsheets
- Magazine and journal articles
- Statistics and surveys
- Government reports
- Literature from special interest groups.

A NOTE ON CRITICAL EVALUATION

Because the information reprinted here is from a number of different sources, readers should bear in mind the origin of the text and whether the source is likely to have a particular bias when presenting information (or when conducting their research). It is hoped that, as you read about the many aspects of the issues explored in this book, you will critically evaluate the information presented.

It is important that you decide whether you are being presented with facts or opinions. Does the writer give a biased or unbiased report? If an opinion is being expressed, do you agree with the writer? Is there potential bias to the 'facts' or statistics behind an article?

ASSIGNMENTS

In the back of this book, you will find a selection of assignments designed to help you engage with the articles you have been reading and to explore your own opinions. Some tasks will take longer than others and there is a mixture of design, writing and research-based activities that you can complete alone or in a group.

FURTHER RESEARCH

At the end of each article we have listed its source and a website that you can visit if you would like to conduct your own research. Please remember to critically evaluate any sources that you consult and consider whether the information you are viewing is accurate and unbiased.

Useful Websites

www.bylinetimes.com

www.edie.net

www.HCMmag.com

www.health.org.uk

www.healthwatch.co.uk

www.historyextra.com

www.ipsos.com

www.lifeline24.co.uk

www.mentalhealth.org.uk

www.nesta.org.uk

www.news-medical.net

www.rcn.org.uk

www.rcpch.ac.uk

www.rsph.org.uk

www.telegraph.co.uk

www.theconversation.com

www.theguardian.com

www.theneweuropean.co.uk

A brief guide to the history of the NHS

Founded to give free healthcare to all, the National Health Service is one of the UK's most beloved institutions. But since it was founded in 1948, it's faced a slew of demanding challenges, from ballooning costs to lethal epidemics.

By Rhiannon Davies

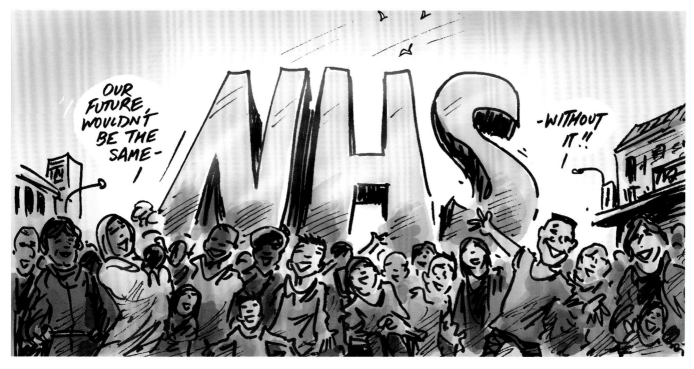

Before the National Health Service (NHS) came into being, Britain's healthcare – and the health of its people – left much to be desired. Pre-Second World War, infectious diseases including diphtheria and tuberculosis were rife, and infant mortality rates were high.

Healthcare was something of a postcode lottery, with those who lived near to institutions like large teaching hospitals in London most likely receiving a higher standard of care than people whose closest port of call was a cottage hospital with few beds. And, of course, people had to pay for their healthcare: in the 1930s, one doctor's visit was approximately three shillings and sixpence – an eye-watering cost that even the middle classes struggled with.

Officials had recommended that a free national health service should be introduced in England as early as 1920. However, it wasn't until 1942 and the release of the Beveridge Report, which set out a system of free healthcare funded by taxes, that it seemed possible such an ambitious project could become a reality.

When did the NHS begin?

On 6 November 1946 Aneurin 'Nye' Bevan, the Minister of Health in Clement Attlee's Labour government, oversaw the passing of legislation that brought the service into being:

the National Health Service Act for England and Wales (there was separate legislation produced for Scotland and Northern Ireland). But, as the country was still economically reeling from the Second World War, the service was not formally founded until 1948.

In the early days, Bevan faced opposition from doctors who were worried that working for the service would limit their independence and hamstring their income. But he eventually persuaded them to join the NHS, later claiming that he had "stuffed their mouths with gold"; he agreed that consultants could keep their private practices and thus retain their financial freedom. On 5 July 1948, the day the NHS officially launched, 85 per cent of doctors had signed up with the service.

Blowing the budget

On that first day, the service took control of 480,000 hospital beds, 125,000 nurses, 5,000 consultants – as well as scores of GPs, opticians, pharmacists, dentists and more.

Setting the budget for such a large service had not been an easy undertaking, and it soon became clear that demand far exceeded supply. The budget for optical services, for example, was 3.5 million for the first year – the actual cost came to a staggering 15 million. And dentists were swamped, too, as Britons who had previously avoided getting their teeth seen to – pre-NHS, people who needed dental work had to travel to a teaching hospital and often pay for services – flocked to see dentists in their droves. In the first year alone, 33 million pairs of dentures were given out. Dentists who had formerly seen 15 or 20 patients a day were now treating up to 100.

Although some people were at first reluctant to use the service, often worrying what their neighbours would think of them for taking something for free, others took advantage of the free assistance on offer. For instance, one doctor was flummoxed by a patient's continual requests for free prescriptions of cotton wool. When he finally asked him what he needed it for, he was stunned to discover the man had been using them to wash his greyhound.

With the budget left in tatters, charges were introduced – the first being for dentures, in the early 1950s. Prescription charges soon followed, initially per prescription before it increased to per item. These charges were later removed by Harold Wilson's Labour government in February 1965, but they gradually crept back in from 1968 onwards. Many exemptions were put in place, though, and a great deal still exist: in 2016, 89.4 per cent of prescriptions were issued free of charge.

Changing attitudes

Throughout the service's history, attitudes towards care – particularly in the case of family planning and mental health – have altered dramatically. Originally family planning was never covered in the service's remit, but when the contraceptive pill was introduced in the 1960s, this was no longer the case. NHS doctors were able to prescribe the pill from the early 1960s onwards – but there was a catch. Only married women were eligible for these prescriptions, and in most cases, they were given out to older women who wanted to stop having children rather than women who didn't want children at all. Unmarried women resorted to subterfuge to secure their access to the pill, slipping on wedding rings in the waiting room to convince their doctors they had husbands. Later in the decade such charades became unnecessary, as the pill was available through the Family Planning Association.

Meanwhile, attitudes to LGBT+ patients came to the fore in the eighties, when the AIDS crisis ravaged England. Following actor Rock Hudson's death from an AIDS-related condition in 1985, UK headlines foretold a plague and stirred up prejudice. The NHS and the department of health were very slow to respond, launching their health campaign about the virus in 1987. With the slogan "Don't die of ignorance", the campaign was meant to raise awareness of the disease and hammer home how dangerous it was: a film commissioned for the campaign prominently featured a tombstone. Contact tracers were also sent out into the community to speak with those who had had relations with AIDS sufferers, and a succession of large-scale campaigns about HIV and safe sex followed.

Treating mental health has changed greatly during the service's history, too. The early NHS inherited a collection of 'asylums' that were in a terrible state. In the 1970s, these asylums were closed down and sold off, and the onus for mental health care was moved towards the community and smaller, local hospitals, with varying levels of success. A raft of new drugs were introduced too, to help treat psychosis and depression, and – particularly in recent years – attitudes towards mental health have largely improved.

Vaccinating the nation

The NHS has carried out several high-profile immunisation drives throughout its history – most notably the vaccination campaigns for polio, measles, and of course the current push to vaccinate the country's population against Covid-19.

Less than a century ago, polio – a debilitating disease that can cause paralysis – was feared across the world. In 1955, a British version of the US vaccine was successfully developed and rolled out across the country. And by 1962, a version of the vaccine that could be administered on a sugar lump was pioneered, which made vaccination even simpler.

However, the public response to the polio vaccination drive was initially rather poor. In the 1950s, epidemics of the disease were breaking out in the Midlands and Northern Ireland. These two spikes in cases helped persuade people to get vaccinated, as well as the surprise death in 1959 of a 29-year-old footballer called Jeff Hall, who had died within a fortnight of being diagnosed with the disease.

Once people were convinced of the need to be vaccinated, the program was rolled out very quickly, and the virus was eventually eradicated in the UK (the last polio outbreak in the country happened in the late 1970s).

But for those who weren't vaccinated in time and who had to be treated by the NHS for polio, their experiences were often horrible. Children recalling their treatments spoke about being kept in iron lungs (machines to assist with breathing which were akin to large metal coffins), and they were rarely allowed to see their parents. Once they were allowed home, they often had to sleep in cold plaster casts and wear callipers (leg braces). However, the polio immunisation drive pales in significance when compared to the race to vaccinate the UK's population against Covid-19 – and treat those who are suffering from its effects. In the words of historian Susan Cohen, "the service has responded absolutely remarkably" to this unprecedented strain on their resources and staff. Cohen says: "They've put their lives on the line to save other people, and that's what the NHS has always been about."

Dr Susan Cohen is a historian with a special interest in British social history.

She was talking to Rhiannon Davies, BBC History Magazine sub editor, on an episode of the HistoryExtra podcast

22 January 2021

Health spending as a share of GDP remains at lowest level in a decade

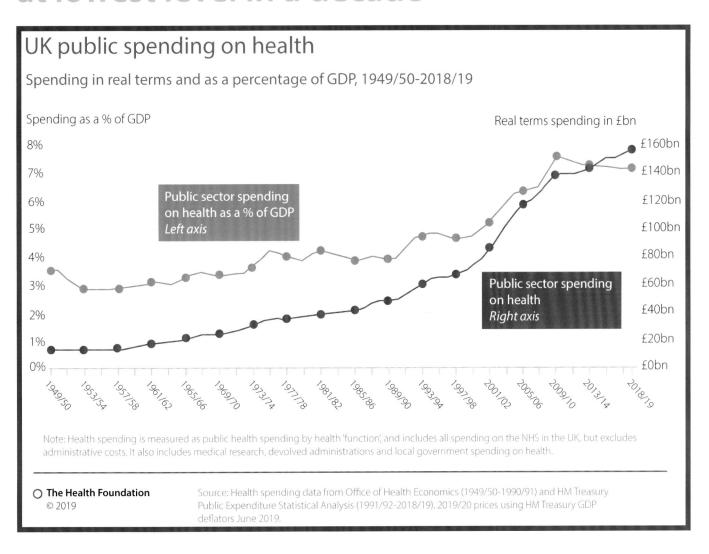

UK public spending on health

Spending in real terms and as a percentage of GDP, 1949/50-2018/19

Spending as a % of GDP

Real terms spending in £bn

Public sector spending on health as a % of GDP
Left axis

Public sector spending on health
Right axis

Note: Health spending is measured as public health spending by health 'function', and includes all spending on the NHS in the UK, but excludes administrative costs. It also includes medical research, devolved administrations and local government spending on health.

The Health Foundation
© 2019

Source: Health spending data from Office of Health Economics (1949/50-1990/91) and HM Treasury Public Expenditure Statistical Analysis (1991/92-2018/19). 2019/20 prices using HM Treasury GDP deflators June 2019.

Key points

◆ As a share of GDP, spending on health in the UK in 2018/19 was roughly the same as it was in 2011/12, and is only marginally above where it was in 2008/09.

◆ This is the result of low growth in health spending, which has risen by 1.6% a year on average since 2011/12, around the same rate as GDP growth.

◆ This is less than half the long-run trend of growth in health spending, which is 3.6% a year in real terms.

In 2018/19 the UK spent around £153bn on health, in 2019/20 prices. This is an increase of 2% compared to the previous year and is ten times more than was spent sixty years earlier, in 1958/59. On average health spending has increased by 3.6% a year over the history of the NHS as a result of the UK's growing population, the increasing prevalence of chronic conditions, and the rising costs of delivering care.

However, over the last decade this growth in health spending has slowed, reaching just 1.6% a year since 2011/12. At that point health spending was 7.3% of GDP, a drop since its highest level of 7.6% in 2009/10. Due to low spending growth since that point the NHS has grown at a similar rate to GDP growth, and it now stands at 7.2% of GDP. In terms of growth as a percentage of GDP, the nine-year period since 2009/10 is the lowest since the first decade of the NHS.

As part of the NHS long term plan a five-year spending settlement has been set out for NHS England. If this spending growth is seen in areas outside of NHS England such as capital spending and the public health grant (and replicated in the devolved administrations) then spending could grow to 7.9% of GDP.

30 July 2019

Public satisfaction with the NHS is high, but waiting times are the public's priority

Latest findings from the Ipsos MORI UK KnowledgePanel show that over two in five expect the general standard of care to get better, and the public's top priority for the NHS is improving waiting times.

By Anna Quigley

New polling by Ipsos MORI, conducted ahead of a webinar co-hosted with the Health Foundation, shows that three-quarters of British adults say that Britain's NHS is one of the best in the world (75% agree), while over six in ten UK adults say they are satisfied with the running of the NHS nowadays (63%).

Pride in the NHS

To what extent do you agree or disagree with each of the following statement?

Britain's National Health Service is one of the best in the world.

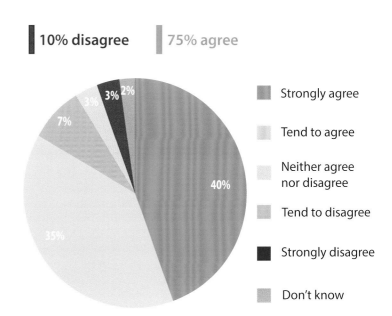

10% disagree   75% agree

- Strongly agree
- Tend to agree
- Neither agree nor disagree
- Tend to disagree
- Strongly disagree
- Don't know

As concern about the pandemic starts to decrease, over two in five people say that they think the standard of care provided by the NHS will get better over the next 12 months (44%), while a third think it will stay the same (35%), and fewer than one in five say it will get worse (17%). The proportion saying that they think it will get worse has decreased since May last year, when it was 25% (45% thought it would get better, while 27% thought it would stay the same).

Expectations of the standard of care

And thinking about the future, do you think the general standard of care provided by the NHS over the next 12 months will get...?

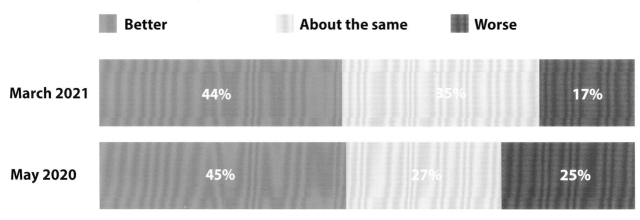

Better   **About the same**   **Worse**

	Better	About the same	Worse
March 2021	44%	35%	17%
May 2020	45%	27%	25%

In particular, the public's top priority for the NHS is improving waiting times. Half say this should be prioritised when the impact of the pandemic has eased, followed by increasing numbers of staff in the NHS (43%), and vaccinating people against COVID-19 (41%). Supporting the wellbeing of NHS staff is important to the public too (38%), as is improving mental health services generally (36%).

Top priorites for the NHS

Thinking about when the impact of the COVID-19 pandemic has eased, when it comes to the NHS, which two or three of the following do you think should be prioritised?

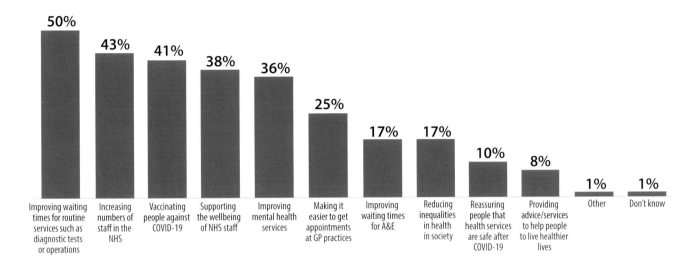

50%	Improving waiting times for routine services such as diagnostic tests or operations
43%	Increasing numbers of staff in the NHS
41%	Vaccinating people against COVID-19
38%	Supporting the wellbeing of NHS staff
36%	Improving mental health services
25%	Making it easier to get appointments at GP practices
17%	Improving waiting times for A&E
17%	Reducing inequalities in health in society
10%	Reassuring people that health services are safe after COVID-19
8%	Providing advice/services to help people to live healthier lives
1%	Other
1%	Don't know

The data shows the difficult task ahead for the NHS. The public recognise the impact of the pandemic on services, with 85% saying that waiting times are longer than before the pandemic. At the same time, six in ten say that current waiting times are unacceptable (61%).

Attitudes towards waiting times

To what extent do you agree or disagree with the following statements?

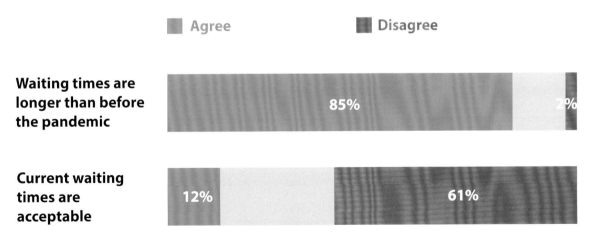

Agree   Disagree

Waiting times are longer than before the pandemic — 85% ... 2%

Current waiting times are acceptable — 12% ... 61%

Anna Quigley, Head of Health and Social Care at Ipsos MORI, said:

"These results show yet again the pride that the public has in the NHS, no doubt bolstered by its work during the pandemic. However, the data also shows the challenges that lie ahead for the NHS in terms of public expectations, at a time when the service is facing a backlog of elective surgery cases, increased demand for mental health services, and the ongoing impact of caring for patients affected by COVID-19".

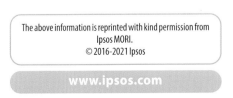

Coronavirus crisis is a turning point for the NHS – for good or bad we just don't know yet

An article from The Conversation.

THE CONVERSATION

By Mark Exworthy, Professor of Health Policy and Management, University of Birmingham

It's hard to imagine anything more transformative for the NHS than the coronavirus crisis. The health and social care system has been making enormous efforts to address the pandemic while the number of deaths continue to rise across the UK. Even now, it is safe to say that 2020 feels like a turning moment in the NHS and beyond.

Our thoughts and efforts may be directed elsewhere at this time but it's also helpful to take stock of the profound changes that are happening and what these may mean for future health service delivery and policy.

NHS staff

We often consider health services in terms of workforce and organisations. In the past few years, NHS staffing has become a significant issue, including a high turnover of senior staff in recent years. Following Brexit uncertainty and the junior doctor strikes in 2016, the Conservatives were re-elected on the promise of "50,000 more nurses" just three months ago. Proposals to restrict (international) migration among "low skilled workers" had presaged further workforce challenges. For some NHS frontline workers, though, visas have now been extended.

The response of staff to COVID-19 has been widely praised by politicians and the general public. Previous cries of support were often rhetorical, but coronavirus has arguably made visible the extent of the professionalism and commitment of staff. If faith in the NHS - the closest thing the British have to a religion as was once said - had been waning, the response of those working in health and social care to tackle coronavirus has surely reaffirmed it.

Flexibility under strain

The NHS has clearly demonstrated incredible flexibility at times of stress. The construction of the Nightingale Hospital in London (and plans for others) illustrates the NHS's (and UK military's) ability to respond. An election promise of 40 "new" hospitals has, however, been pushed back.

A focus on building new hospitals captures political attention and tends to increase a fixation on acute services (rather than primary or social care). But staffing roles are being rapidly reshaped by coronavirus responses; the boundaries between and within clinical professions (especially in clinical settings) are being blurred in ways that would have seemed unimaginable a short while ago.

Staff shortages and staff sickness mean clinical staff are also having to work in unfamiliar ways to respond to the volume of coronavirus cases, for example eye surgeons working in intensive care units. This also entails a shift in the balance between specialist and generalist practice, which will, in turn, determine how centralised services will become.

Other impacts

There has been much less focus on the impact and consequences of coronavirus for social care and its staff. For example, the discharge of patients from hospital into settings such as nursing homes, where protective equipment is less widespread, is unknown. The short and long-term effect on health and care staff wellbeing is also likely to be significant during a period of new roles and high stress.

The NHS has also been running at an increasing tempo in recent years, with service very near full capacity. Targets have been missed, for example, on A&E waiting times for some time (70% of patients at major emergency departments were seen within four hours, against a standard of 95%), while the number of beds in English NHS hospitals has halved in the last 30 years (from 299,000 in 1987-88 to 141,000 in 2018-19). Likewise, the UK has 2.8 doctors per 1,000 population compared to 4.0 in Italy or 4.3 in Germany.

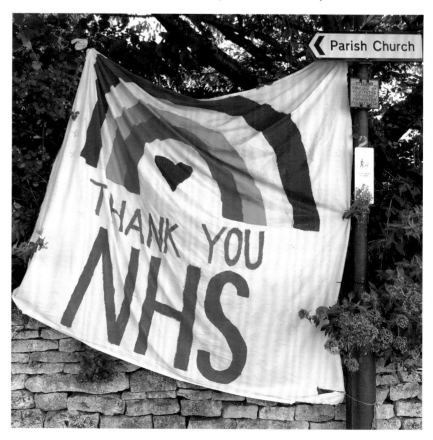

Operational shifts

The NHS had entered the pandemic phase in an exposed state. As financial deficits grew, so-called "winter pressures" began affecting the NHS all year round (though this winter was a mild one). Nonetheless, operational responses have been swift and/or profound:

⬥ Coronavirus has rapidly increased the spread and reach of telephone and video consultations in primary and secondary care. It's highly unlikely that normal (non-digital) service will be resumed – with possible increases in demand (video consultations don't necessarily reduce demand).

⬥ The private sector has previously been used to alleviate pressures, such as waiting times for elective procedures. But this time the two sectors have been more closely bound, including the private sector providing more extensive cancer care.

⬥ The commissioning role of the NHS has effectively been centralised. Clinical Commissioning Groups, which planned and commissioned health services for local areas, have been taken over by NHS England. Many had already been merged or amalgamated, and could spell the end of this commissioning experiment. Long-term plans now look redundant.

⬥ A period of incremental and transitional change in the NHS is over; coronavirus has instead introduced dramatic and transformational change. To navigate this, the NHS is relying on the resilience and ingenuity of staff, but the high turnover of senior staff and in turn the loss of organisational memory will hamper this. In a post-COVID era, public finances will also be extremely strained, possibly heralding a new era of austerity, despite the government recently "writing off" £13 billion of historic NHS providers' debts. And the NHS still has the impact of Brexit to negotiate.

Coronavirus presents an immediate crisis for the NHS but there will be longer-term changes that, for now, remain unknown. What we do know is that 2020 will register as a seminal turning point in British health policy.

This article was co-authored with Charles Tallack, a health analyst from the Health Foundation.

21 April 2021

Young doctors wanting to work part-time 'threatens NHS staffing crisis'

During the pandemic, virtual triage and consultations have sped up treatments and reduced the number of unnecessary in-person interactions.

By Joe Pinkstone, Science Correspondent

More than half of trainees (56 per cent) working for the NHS are considering only working part-time hours, according to figures released by a royal college.

A fifth of doctors already work part-time and this trend looks likely to increase in popularity, according to a survey from the Royal College of Physicians (RCP).

It also revealed that more than a quarter of senior consultant physicians are expected to retire in the next three years, with many expected to depart in the next 18 months.

The findings have caused alarm that an already substantial NHS staffing crisis is only going to worsen as the UK moves into a post-Covid-19 world.

The data comes from an RCP poll of 1,523 medics commissioned to celebrate the 73rd birthday of the NHS.

Virtual triage and consultations

More than 60 per cent – rising to 72 per cent for trainees – of respondents said they want opportunities for remote IT access, online meetings and remote working in the future.

Remote working has been a huge success during the Covid-19 pandemic, with virtual triage and consultations speeding up treatments and helping to reduce wait times, while also reducing the number of unnecessary in-person interactions.

One example is abortions, where legislation introduced in April 2020 as a result of the pandemic allowed women to take both doses of their medication at home, instead of in a clinic.

They were also able to have both their consultations done remotely and, as a result, more abortions were conducted quicker than at any point since records began.

"If a majority of trainees coming into the system are keen to work part-time, we need to find a way to make that happen to keep attracting people into the profession and retaining them," said Andrew Goddard, president of the RCP.

"The NHS has recognised that and wants to offer flexible working – but it is stuck in a true Catch-22 situation where it cannot do the very thing needed to attract more staff because it doesn't have enough staff at the moment."

NHS bosses have also used the anniversary to address the increasing shortage of staff.

An open letter was penned by the country's most senior health professionals, including the chief nursing officer, Ruth May, Professor Stephen Powis, national medical director, and Suzanne Rastrick, the NHS's chief allied health professions officer.

"With the pandemic response entering the recovery phase and as we tackle new challenges like long Covid, the NHS is looking for more talented and committed staff who will go the extra mile for patients and their families," it reads.

"As the NHS marks its 73rd birthday, we are asking young people wondering what path to take, and anyone thinking about a career change, to consider joining us."

However, low pay is viewed as a significant barrier in allowing the health service to meet this demand.

Unite, which has 100,000 members in the health service, has said the one per cent pay rise for healthcare workers is insufficient and should be increased.

Last week, senior medics at the British Medical Association said they would consider taking industrial action if the figure was not increased to around four per cent.

This echoes the severe discontent of the Royal College of Nursing, which is said to be considering strike action. The RCN had asked for a 12.5 per cent pay rise for nurses.

"The NHS has an estimated 100,000 vacancies, including 40,000 nursing posts – and one way to tackle this ever-growing problem is to substantially boost the pay of NHS staff," said Colenzo Jarrett-Thorpe, Unite national officer for health.

"If the new Health and Social Care Secretary Sajid Javid is unable to obtain a lot more cash from the Chief Secretary to the Treasury Stephen Barclay for the health service, the NHS will be a pale shadow of the great Covid-fighting health service we know and love in five years' time."

Andrew Goddard, president of the RCP, said: "If we do not address this problem [of staff shortages], we will have much less to celebrate in future."

The RCP said medical school places need to be doubled to avoid medical staff shortages worsening in the future.

Meanwhile, there needs to be increased funding for social care and action to address health inequalities to reduce demands on the NHS, it said.

5 July 2021

UK has highest health worker COVID deaths in Europe and third highest worldwide

Stephen Colegrave investigates why Medscape indicates the UK has had so many more health worker deaths than elsewhere.

By Stephen Colegrave

The Medscape memorial figures for COVID-19 deaths provides a poignant insight into the magnitude of health worker deaths compared to the rest of the world. The gap between the UK's number of deaths compared with any other European country has increased since Byline Times looked at these figures last year. The only other two countries anywhere near Britain's high levels of health worker deaths are Italy and Spain with 28% and 46% fewer deaths respectively.

When size of population is taken into account, the UK has the third highest death rate worldwide with nearly three times as many health worker deaths in comparison than the USA, even though most of these were on Trump's watch. Only El Salvador and Mexico have worse figures.

The UK's appalling figures are an indictment of the Government's failure to provide adequate personal protective (PPE) clothing for health workers. This was depicted most dramatically by the image of nurses in Northwick Park Hospital trying to make their own PPE out of

bin liners in April 2020 because nothing else was available. According to the Daily Mirror, a few weeks later they tested positive for COVID-19.

This was followed by the farce of PPE flown in from Turkey by the RAF including 400,000 much needed gowns accompanied by triumphant and bellicose promises by Matt Hancock, much of which proved to be sub-standard as the Metro reported on 7 May 2020.

"The vital PPE was flown into the UK by the RAF as Britain's essential heath and care workers continued to risk their lives without proper protection. But the gowns never made it to the frontline and are instead being kept inside a Government warehouse near Heathrow airport after falling short of UK standards".

There was certainly no lack on money spent of PPE, more than £36 billion so far, so why have our health care workers been so poorly protected?

Since then the Government has been determined to deflect any criticism about the inadequacy of its provision of PPE

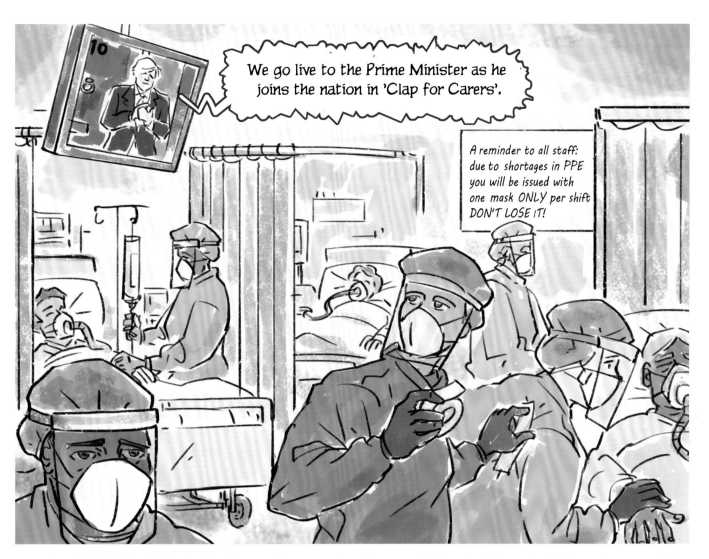

even though Public Health England guidance often seemed to have been driven by availability rather than international best practice and often fell short of WHO guidelines. This has been highlighted by campaigning group EveryDoctor UK.

Last November, Labour leader Keir Starmer had the temerity to question the Prime Minister over the adequacy of PPE, who confidently declared that "99.5% of the 32 billion items of personal protective equipment conformed entirely to our clinical needs."

This was at odds with the evidence given to the Public Accounts Committee by DHSC permanent secretary Sir Chris Wormald that 2.9 billion items of PPE costing £1.5 billion were inadequate for use in a clinical setting, as reported in Byline Times last week.

As well as PPE, in the first wave of the pandemic, testing of health workers was slow to be implemented at scale and consistently failed to meet targets.

This not only put health care workers' lives at risks but also many patients and most devastatingly led to elderly patients being discharged into care homes with deadly results.

Indeed, at the time Department of Health and Social Care guidance stated that "negative tests are not required prior to transfers/admissions into the care home". This guidance and the general lack of testing led to many care worker deaths as well as care home residents becoming the population with the most COVID-19 deaths in the country.

The worst thing about these tragic figures is an overriding sense that many deaths could have been avoided if health workers had not been let down by inadequacies in policy and implementation of PPE and testing by a Government that is determined never to admit its mistakes.

"The UK healthcare worker death toll is devastating," EveryDoctor CEO Dr Julia Patterson told Byline Times. The organisation represents the concerns of NHS doctors and were co-claimants in the Good Law Project's case against the Government over PPE procurement.

"Many of these frontline workers were provided with no PPE at all during the first wave of COVID-19," she continued. "These workers were unprotected as they saved lives, and the UK government have failed to take responsibility. NHS staff need better PPE; the COVID 19 case numbers are rising and every frontline health and social care worker should be provided with respirator masks because COVID-19 is airborne. This situation must never happen again."

15 June 2021

NHS drops from first to fourth among rich countries' healthcare systems

Thinktank says longer wait for treatment since Covid pandemic is main reason, in study of 11 countries.

By Denis Campbell, Health Policy Editor

The NHS has lost its prestigious ranking as the best health system in a study of 11 rich countries by an influential US thinktank.

The UK has fallen from first to fourth in the Commonwealth Fund's latest analysis of the performance of the healthcare systems in the nations it studied.

Norway, the Netherlands and Australia now provide better care than the UK, it found. The findings are a blow to the NHS, which had been the top-rated system in the thinktank's two previous reports in 2017 and 2014. The US had by far the worst-rated system, despite spending the most on care.

The Washington-based Commonwealth Fund blamed the NHS's slip down its league table on the delays patients face in accessing care and treatment, lack of investment in the service and poverty.

"According to this report, our previously world-beating health service is at risk of moving to the middle of the pack, largely due to growing delays across the system in people's ability to access care quickly," said Siva Anandaciva, the chief analyst at the King's Fund, the leading UK health thinktank.

"We can't brush this under the carpet as being solely a consequence of the impact of the pandemic on patients, staff and services. Even before Covid, waiting lists for treatment were already sizeable after a decade of stalling funding and a growing workforce crisis.

"As Covid put the NHS under unprecedented pressure, the waiting list for routine NHS care has ballooned to levels not seen since the early 2000s. Whilst the NHS is doing its best to keep services running, increasing demand for hospital, mental health and GP services means the whole health and care system is now facing a capacity crunch," he added.

Eric Schneider, lead author of the Commonwealth Fund's Mirror, Mirror 2021 report, said the UK had scored lower marks compared with 2017 on three of the five domains its panel of experts used: access to care; care processes, which look at the co-ordination of treatment and how well patients are involved; and equity, or the ability to obtain healthcare regardless of income.

He pinpointed the time taken to access care in the UK as a key factor in its ranking. "For example, nearly 60% of adults in the UK found it somewhat or very difficult to obtain after-hours care, one of the highest rates among the countries surveyed," he said.

The study also found that while 78% of Britons in 2017 said that their regular doctor always or often answered a query on the day they posed it, just 65% did so this year.

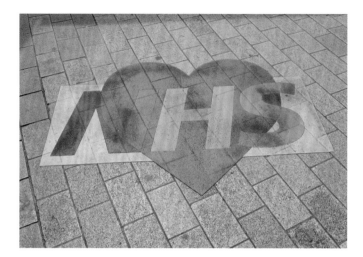

Similarly, while 57% in 2017 said they saw a doctor or nurse on the same or next day the last time they sought care, that has fallen to 52%.

In addition, just 33% of patients said that they got counselling or treatment for mental health problems when they sought help from a specialist in psychological or psychiatric illness – a new indicator that the thinktank had not previously analysed. The NHS was the second worst performer of the 11 countries on that criterion, just ahead of France.

As well as being ranked fourth overall the UK was also ranked fourth out of 11 for access to care, administrative efficiency and equity, and fifth for care processes but just ninth for health care outcomes, which measures how well patients recover after undergoing medical treatment.

Asked to explain the NHS's decline relative to the other nations, Schneider added: "We know that reported experiences of access, co-ordination and engagement can deteriorate over time if budgets are cut. The UK has been a remarkably lean spender among high-income countries while nevertheless maintaining a very high ranking."

NHS England declined to comment. A Department of Health and Social Care spokesperson said: "We are committed to making sure the NHS has everything it needs to continue providing excellent care to the public, as we tackle the backlogs that have built up.

"We gave the NHS a historic settlement in 2018, which will see its budget rise by £33.9bn by 2023/24, and we have provided an extra £92bn to support health and care services throughout the pandemic."

4 August 2021

Twin crisis of access and affordability calls for a radical rethink of NHS dentistry

New data indicates the dental crisis shows no signs of slowing, with four in five people (80%) struggling to access timely care during the last COVID-19 lockdown.

Access to NHS dental care continues to be a problem for people across England, with Healthwatch recording a 22% rise in calls and complaints about dentistry between January and March 2021.

Our review of 1,375 people's experiences shared with Healthwatch found a lack of consistency across the country when it comes to accessing a dental appointment. Whilst some people were asked to wait an unreasonable time of up to three years for an NHS appointment, those able to afford private care could get an appointment within a week.

High cost of dental care

Whilst some people were charged £400 to get one tooth out, an individual reported being asked to pay over £7,000 for their dentures privately.

But private treatment is not an option for everyone, with many people now struggling to pay even for NHS treatment.

A poll of 2,019 adults commissioned by us found 61% of respondents felt that NHS dental treatments were expensive.[1] The poll, which looked at people's experiences of NHS dentistry during the pandemic and how it has impacted their future habits, found the following:

People's experiences of NHS dental charges

- Over a quarter (27%) of respondents said they either struggle to pay or avoid dental treatments altogether because they cannot afford the costs.

- About one in three (30%) have reported they felt pressured into paying private fees to get all the dental treatment they needed. And nearly two in five (39%) reported that they had been charged extra for their NHS treatments.

- Almost a quarter (23%) feel they will now visit the dentist only when they need treatment, despite clinical guidelines recommending regular dental check-ups to keep people's mouths healthy.

- Demographic groups who have been affected the most by the lack of NHS dental appointments and NHS dental fees include people on low incomes and those from ethnic minority groups – the same groups who have been worst hit by the COVID-19 pandemic.

Calling for equitable and affordable dental care

Reform of dentistry has been underway since 2009. Earlier this year, it was announced that NHS England would be taking over the process from the Department of Health and Social Care, but reform plans have yet to be announced.

In a recent report on the future of the NHS, the Lancet Commission stressed 'an absence of affordability is a major barrier to dental care' and suggested an abolition of patients' co-payments to access and receive dental care.

We call for greater ambition and urgency from NHS dental reform plans to create more equitable and affordable dental care.

Imelda Redmond CBE, National Director of Healthwatch England, said: "The twin crisis of access and affordability hitting NHS dentistry means many people are not able to access timely care – and the poorest are hardest hit. Those human stories show that oral health is a social justice and equity issue.

Reform of dental contracts needs to be a matter of urgency for this Government. New arrangements should include making access to NHS dental services equal and affordable for everyone, regardless of where people live, their income and ethnicity. Failing to act now will result in long-term harm

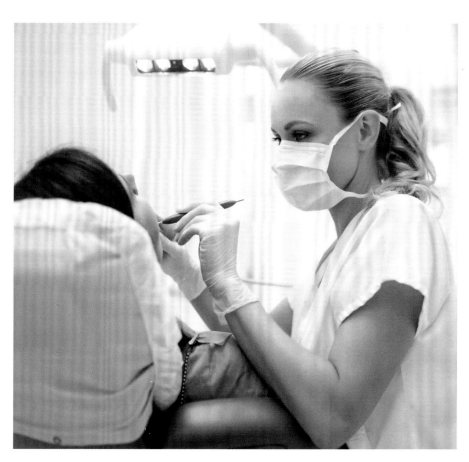

for thousands of people, putting even greater pressure on the already overstretched healthcare system."

– Imelda Redmond CBE, National Director of Healthwatch England

The impact on individuals

Gwen Leeming from Brighton has been suffering over the last couple of years with bad infections in two of her back teeth. She would take paracetamol and saltwater to help her sore mouth and throat. After being told by her NHS dentist last autumn they are only open for private patients, it took her six months to see an NHS surgical dentist.

"I am a 72-year-old who has worked and paid National Insurance for over 50 years, so I can't get health insurance any longer. As I live on limited income, which is supplemented by housing benefit, I can't afford extra costs like private dental care.

"I'm one of the many victims of our broken dental care system. It particularly is failing older patients who suffered (indeed still suffer) from the impact of 1960's school dentists."

Income and regional disparities

Almost twice as many people from lower socio-economic groups (SEG) D and E struggle or can't afford to pay NHS dental charges (37%) than people from the higher socioeconomic group, A, (19%). As a result, people from SEG D and E are also twice as likely to avoid dental care due to affordability issues.

People living in the North East of England are the most likely to avoid NHS dental treatment due to costs (13%), compared with just one in 30 (3%) who live in the South West. Despite this, people in the North East have been charged for NHS dental treatments the most (29%), while people in the South West were charged the least (13%).

People from ethnic minority groups

Just over a quarter of people from ethnic minority communities (26%) reported they would go to the dentist for regular check-ups, compared to two in five (41%) of White people. The survey also found that people aged over 55 from ethnic minority groups who are on low incomes were six times more likely to report avoiding dental treatments due to costs than their White counterparts.

1 - The online poll was carried out by Yonder Data Solutions from February 19-25, 2021, and received responses from 2,019 adults (aged 18+) based in England.

24 May 2021

Healthcare systems around the world

There are many philosophies shaping healthcare services around the world, and this article glances at some prominent examples. This may help understand why different countries experience healthcare differently.

By Dr. Liji Thomas, MD. *Reviewed by* Sophia Coveney, B.Sc.

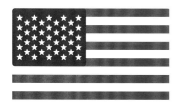

Healthcare in the USA

The USA does not have a universal, free healthcare program, unlike most other developed countries. Instead, in line with the free-market-virtue mindset, most Americans are served by a mix of publicly and privately funded programs and healthcare systems.

Most hospitals and clinics are privately owned, with about 60% being non-profits, and another fifth being for-profit facilities. Coverage by federal and state programs is partial, and most insured Americans have employment-based private insurance.

Group plans funded by the employer cover about 150 million Americans.

Private insurance

These include health maintenance organizations (HMOs), which are networks of providers. Insured patients see a primary care physician (PCP), who refers them to a specialist if necessary.

A more popular option is to use preferred provider organizations (PPOs), which allow patients to see external providers, choose their PCPs, and see a specialist without a PCP referral provided the former is willing.

These are now used by over 55% of insured employees, compared to 25% in HMOs or point-of-service (POS) plans.

With POS plans, patients must have a PCP in the provider network, but can go out of the network for a fee.

Federal insurance

The Indian Health Services and Veteran Health Administration provide care for Native Americans and military veterans, respectively. The Military Health System, operated by the Department of Defense, provides paid care to serving military personnel.

Publicly funded insurance

Public spending accounts for at least half of all healthcare expenditure, while third-party payers pay only 27%.

About a third of the population is covered by three publicly funded programs – Medicare, for people above 65 years and some disabled people, Medicaid, for those living in poverty, and the Children's Health Insurance programs, which cover children from families that are not eligible for Medicaid, at above 300 percent of the Federal Poverty Level (FPL).

The ACA act of 2010 ("Obamacare"), which was enacted in 2010, revamped health insurance. It created health insurance marketplaces, which cover about 17 million Americans. However, these plans are often small, exclusive, and restricted in provider choice.

At the same time, the expansion of Medicaid under the ACA act has possibly saved many lives at less than $900,000 per life saved, vs $7.6 million under other public insurance plans.

The good and the bad

Among 11 high-income countries, the US healthcare system is the most expensive, with 17% of the GDP being spent on healthcare in 2018. Many American health indicators far surpass world standards.

Its rate of specialized scans (computerized tomography – CT – and MRI) – are among the highest in the world, at double the OECD average. So is its utilization of hip replacements, influenza vaccines, and breast cancer screenings.

However, among developed countries, the American system is among the least accessible, efficient and equitable. The number of physicians, and rate of physician visits, is among the lowest. Ethnic and disadvantaged social groups suffer massive inequalities.

About 14% of Americans (over 27 million) were uninsured against illness at the end of 2018, causing an estimated 60,000 avoidable deaths. High medical costs have led to bankruptcy for a fourth of senior citizens, says an earlier study. Preventable and lifestyle conditions such as obesity, hypertension and diabetes are rampant: this indicates poor access to primary care and primary prevention of disease, compared to its peers.

Meanwhile, US suicide rates are highest among all members of the Organization for Economic Co-operation and Development (OECD).

Overall, the US healthcare system allows providers to inflate prices and expensive services, but poorly compensates essential services such as primary care and behavioral advice. It also draws healthcare services away from rural and poor communities. Nonetheless, the US leads in medical innovation, boasting many of the world's leading hospitals. For those who can pay, it provides high-quality care.

COVID-19 response

Even though the US healthcare system serves 4% of the world's population, a quarter of global COVID-19 cases and a fifth of global COVID-19 deaths occurred here. The reasons are not primarily related to the healthcare system, however.

Rather, they include a disjointed, reluctant and often contradictory public health response to the pandemic, driven by political apathy toward the virus threat.

There is no central command and control for healthcare in the country: this obstructs infection spread control.

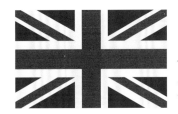

UK healthcare system

The UK healthcare system covers the whole population via the National Health Service (NHS), which is 79% publicly financed from taxes, and operated by the Department of Health. About 20% is paid for by national insurance, and private patients and copayments make up the rest.

NHS England supervises and funds local Clinical Commissioning Groups. These provide comprehensive care, including preventive screening programs and vaccinations, inpatient and outpatient care in hospitals, maternity care, mental health care and palliative care.

Like the USA, the UK has public, private profit and nonprofit hospitals. The first type is operated as hospital trusts or foundation trusts, in three tiers: community hospitals, district hospitals, and regional-level hospitals. Dedicated hospitals offer specialized treatment.

General practitioners (GPs) offer primary care to locals through their practices. Many such practices are overtaxed: one alternative is registration-free walk-in centers. GPs refer patients as necessary for secondary care.

All residents of England, as well as anyone with a European Health Insurance Card, are entitled to NHS care: primary care is mostly free. Others receive emergency or infection-selective treatment.

Patients in the NHS can choose a hospital and specialist. Currently, 12% of the population also opts for private health insurance, mainly to avoid the waiting period for elective care, to have a choice of specialists, and better facilities.

Private hospitals typically offer specialized treatments, such as bariatric surgery, and do not offer trauma care, emergency services or intensive care.

The UK spends about a tenth of its GDP on healthcare, with almost 80% being spent on the NHS.

Unlike the American healthcare system, the NHS's administrative spending is only 16% of healthcare costs.

The good and the bad

Universal free healthcare is widely considered to be good for the country, health-wise as well as economically.

The UK NHS provides free healthcare for all and higher life expectancy than in the USA, at half the cost. Patient satisfaction is relatively high, at 61%, compared to 29% in the US. Taxes for healthcare may appear higher but are actually equivalent to the total medical expenses in the US. Moreover, drugs are cheaper, and there are no surprise medical costs.

Austerity cuts have led to a reluctance to recruit staff and to upgrade equipment, which may eventually affect the quality of care. Waiting times for consultations and surgeries are long.

A third issue is health tourism, where non-residents exploit the NHS to get high-quality medical care at a lower cost than is available where they live, but without a corresponding contribution through taxes.

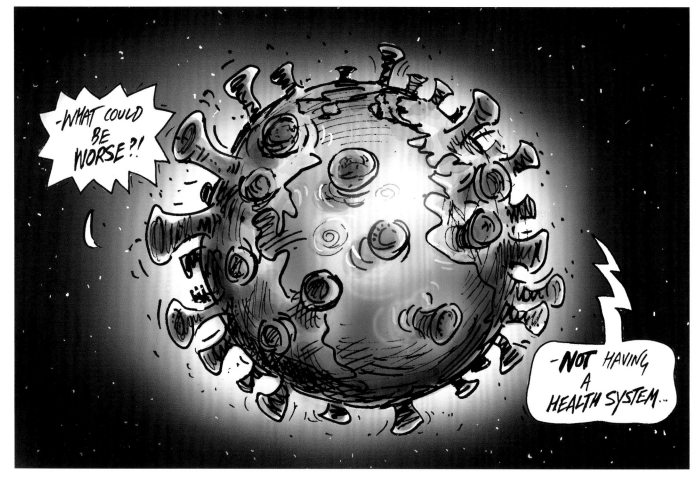

Ethnic minorities and the poor face inequality in the healthcare system. Social care measures need to be implemented.

COVID-19 response

When the pandemic hit the UK, the government built seven temporary hospitals to cope with the sudden demand.

Case finding, contact tracing and isolation were woefully inadequate, allowing community spread to occur and forcing local authorities to take over.

Routine medical care was affected by the pandemic. Patients avoided the emergency department for fear of infection. At least 160,000 patients waited a year for diagnoses, vs the standard 18 weeks. Restoration of this standard may take years.

Mental health care, already pressured, is under massively increased stress, with an estimated 10 million new patients influenced by the pandemic.

Many staff were infected or exposed to infection: to compensate, others have been asked to forego or limit planned leave.

The new spike of cases in 2021 has caused more hospitalizations than at the peak in 2020.

Additionally, the NHS is required to ensure vaccination of the whole country. Thirdly, it has to arrange long-term follow-up services for people with long COVID.

In order to restructure the NHS to meet all these needs, three areas must be prioritized – capacity, resources and public health.

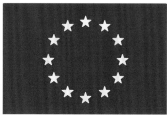

Healthcare in the European Union

Each country in the EU has its own healthcare system. However, EU members generally share the same goal as the UK model.

All healthcare systems in Europe automatically include all citizens irrespective of paying capacity. Secondly, all are mostly funded by taxes paid by the employer and by the public. Healthcare is free, except for some elective and specialist services.

Three models

There are fundamentally three models at work within the EU: single-payer, socialized, and privatized-regulated.

In a single-payer system, the government provides universal insurance or coverage, but the actual care is by private practices and hospitals.

Individuals may opt for additional private insurance to cover services that are not covered by public healthcare, but not for those already available. The payment for such providers may be fee-for-service, or capitation, based on the number of patients enrolled.

More recently, lump-sum payments have been adopted to cover all services per year per person enrolled. However, fee-for-service tends to encourage excessive use of manpower and capital resources.

Hospital funds are allocated as diagnosis-related groups (DRGs), per-diem, or as lump-sum payments for all services.

The socialized system is one where the government both provides insurance and runs the hospitals. It is thus the only health insurance provider. The NHS is a version of this model, which is also used in France, Italy, Norway and Sweden.

Patients may opt for supplemental private insurance, to get services not supplied within the public health service, or to see doctors not employed by this service.

France, cited by some as having among the best healthcare systems in the world, has a significant private healthcare system as well as statutory health insurance, offering a wide choice of coverage.

However, recent amendments to the law made it mandatory for employees to pay half of the insurance sponsored by their employers. This is especially so for dental and vision expenses, not covered by the state health insurance.

This system strongly resembles the American Medicare, Medicaid and Veteran Affairs schemes.

The privatized but regulated healthcare systems within the EU are exemplified by Germany. Here, though all citizens earning below a threshold must take health insurance, their unemployed spouses and dependants are also covered without any extra cost.

Above this threshold, employees may buy private insurance. However, other than self-employed and government servants, most people prefer not to.

In Switzerland and the Netherlands, health insurance is mandatory and provided exclusively by private providers. The government subsidizes the premiums through taxes, making it possible for even low-earning citizens to afford health insurance.

All insurers are legally required to accept any applicant. This costs the patient much less than it would in the US, the system is easier to navigate, and the coinsurance is capped at a reasonable ceiling.

Thus, European healthcare provides primary and some secondary medical care, with some places allowing private companies to sponsor more insurance for their employees.

Privatized programs allow for specialized care, cut down the waiting time for a procedure, or expand the patient's choices.

The EU average for healthcare expenditure is about 8% of the GDP, but Cyprus and Latvia are at 3.5%, with other East European nations at 5%. Public spending in this sector typically makes up about 15% of the total government budget.

The good and the bad

Most EU members enjoy the approval of the majority of their people for their healthcare systems, with less than 5% of people in four-fifths of European countries reporting unmet needs.

National health systems tend to control costs better. The introduction of internal markets may increase the healthcare economy and efficiency.

Nonetheless, funding pressures are likely to go up as patients expect more advanced treatments and as technology develops. The graying of Europe may impede fund flows to these programs, given that about 70% of the funding comes from the public sector in most countries.

At the same time, aging is associated with different patterns of disease, typically conditions that are both preventable and care-intensive. As age increases, however, social welfare tends to absorb more of the costs.

Audits of spending efficiency will be crucial to enhancing the spending power of each euro. "The OECD estimates that one fifth of health expenditure makes little or no contribution to improving people's health."

Inequalities in health status and inequity in healthcare finance and delivery continue to plague the system in many EU nations.

COVID-19 response

While many countries set up smoothly functioning mechanisms to deal with the emerging pandemic, the EU was, generally, unprepared. The stockpiles of equipment, medicines and ventilators were inadequate in many places.

This hampered these countries from buying testing kits and setting up contact tracing, for example, early in the pandemic, which further slowed down virus containment efforts.

Crisis management plans fell short of reality, forcing healthcare staff to improvise and innovate, as well as overwork, to compensate. The need to share resources, and hospital capacity, internationally, could also be significant.

Thus, logistics, preparedness, coordination, and continuing with routine healthcare, are areas that need future improvement.

Healthcare systems in Asia

Asian healthcare systems are a mélange of public and privately managed programs.

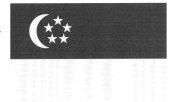

Singapore

Singapore uses the 3Ms system: a public statutory insurance system, MediShield Life for large hospital bills, and some high-end outpatient treatments as well, but not primary care, or specialist care at the outpatient level. The premiums are subsidized to help even low-earning people to pay them, and working-age people pay more to allow older people to enjoy lower premiums.

A compulsory national health savings account called MediSave helps pay for hospital care and some outpatient treatments. MediFund is a social welfare program for poor citizens who cannot pay for out-of-pocket expenses even with MediSave.

Thus, the government, healthcare providers, and patients all share the responsibility for healthcare coverage – a multipayer financing system. While competition and market forces enhance the quality of healthcare, the government strictly regulates the costs when they begin to rise beyond affordable rates.

The Ministry of Health also plans for workforce strength, training and land allotment for healthcare facilities, along with preventive health interventions. The system's centralized nature keeps administrative costs low and simplifies procedures.

Singapore spends about 4.5% of its GDP on healthcare, about 40% by the government, with 30% being out-of-pocket expenses.

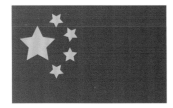

China

China has almost universal publicly funded medical insurance, with urban employees enrolled in employment-based programs. Others enroll voluntarily, for basic subsidized medical insurance. Comprehensive healthcare is covered, but deductibles and copayments apply. There is also a ceiling on reimbursement.

For-profit private insurance is also available for services not covered by public insurance. Patients share costs for physician visits, inpatient care and prescription drugs, which are uncapped.

China spends about 6.6% of its GDP on healthcare, with 28% being funded by central and local governments, 28% out-of-pocket, and 44% by public or private insurance, and social health donations. These form part of a medical assistance program for the poor.

Wide inequalities in public health services have been reported. Most residents feel that their insurance is as helpful, at least, as the basic public health services.

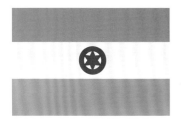

India

India provides universal free outpatient and inpatient care at government clinics and hospitals. States are in charge of organizing their healthcare services.

However, government facilities are notoriously understaffed and ill-equipped, so that most people pay out-of-pocket for private healthcare. The National Health Protection Scheme (Ayushman Bharat-Pradhan Mantri Jan Arogya Yojana, or PM-JAY) was recently launched to attempt to address this: it supersedes the earlier under-performing National Health Insurance Program (Rashtriya Swasthya Bima Yojana, or RSBY).

The PM-JAY program is financed by taxes and enables free secondary and tertiary care at private hospitals. PM-JAY envisages grassroots Health and Wellness Centers while providing cashless hospital care for the 40% of people (approximately 100 million) who live below the poverty line.

Government workers and most formal employees have their own health insurance schemes. A few private health insurance providers also exist, with limited uptake. Less than 40% of Indians are insured.

The situation is worsened by the poor quality of public healthcare services and the shortage of doctors and equipment. Corruption, as in many developing countries, along with accessibility issues, exacerbates these drawbacks.

India spends less than 4% of its GDP on healthcare, with a quarter being funded by the public sector. Out-of-pocket payments at private hospitals make up 75% of the total expenditure, in stark contrast to other poor countries.

COVID-19 response

The overall strategy in east Asia's advanced economies was to suppress the spread of the virus using conventional containment measures.

Careful case tracking, contact tracing, and quarantine helped contain the virus in Singapore, Hong Kong and South Korea, for instance.

Even in less economically advanced countries like India, the Philippines, and Vietnam, public health education and preexisting community values proved useful. These commonly shared values allowed people to take more easily to non-pharmaceutical interventions (NPIs) such as masking up, staying at home, and social distancing.

In India, the lockdown was a key weapon against the spread of the virus. This was coupled with a ramping up of production of personal protective equipment, ventilators and testing kits.

Yet, extreme and widespread poverty, weak healthcare systems and the high population density make tracking and countering the pandemic a difficult task in India, as in other developing Asian countries.

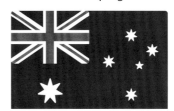

Healthcare systems in Australia

Australia has a tax-funded universal free public health insurance program, called Medicare. All citizens get free care for public and many physician services and drugs at public hospitals.

About 50% of Australian citizens also take out private insurance to pay for private hospital care or dental care. This is encouraged by the government, and high-income families pay a tax penalty for not buying private insurance.

The total expenditure on healthcare is about 10% of GDP, with 67% being from the public sector. It is jointly run by federal, state and territorial governments, and is among the best in the world.

Pros and cons

While free universal care is an undoubted advantage, funding may be challenging as the population ages, reducing tax inflow. Meanwhile, medical technology costs go up, making it difficult to keep up.

There is a disparity in access and care quality between the non-indigenous and the aboriginal population. Research is not well-aligned with national priorities. Urbanization continues to pose an obstacle to healthy living.

COVID-19 response

The Australian response to the pandemic included building transparency between the government and citizens, to ensure public trust. This in turn resulted in a high level of compliance to lockdowns, masking up and quarantine, as well as rapid testing.

Secondly, the decision-making process was driven by reliable data interpreted by experts and performed in an agile and iterative manner. Both political and public health leaders were seen to be cooperating and trustworthy.

Thirdly, the pandemic response was based on a collaboration across health and economic boundaries. The public health response was both willing and strong, which certainly helped to achieve the goal of virus containment.

This resulted in low mortality and infection rates, as well as a rapidly rebounding economy. Localized outbreaks still occur, and are handled on a crisis level. This has come at the cost of many stranded Australians abroad who cannot return home due to the cap on the number of returning passengers.

Healthcare systems in South America

While medical services tend to be cheaper here, they are also universal and publicly funded in countries like Chile and Columbia. As a result, medical tourism has boomed in these places.

Healthcare systems have progressed since the time when only employees in the formal labor market received public health insurance, to which employers, employees and government contributed.

The rest of the people relied on fragmentary services by the Ministry of Health, the church, and charitable or philanthropic organizations. The rich had private health care. The poor had almost nothing.

A few examples

Colombia

Colombia is a success story in South American healthcare. It covers almost 97% of its population by mandatory universal health insurance. All citizens have access to the same healthcare services, with only 14% out-of-pocket spending. This is lower than that in many OECD countries.

The health system is financed through taxes and employment insurance and fully subsidizes the poor. Both public and private insurers are involved, and providers also belong to both public and private sectors, with a healthy competition between the two.

The FOSYGA; Solidarity and Guarantee Fund, is based on cross-subsidies between rich and poor, young and old, and healthy vs sick.

Participants may choose their provider within their network, and receive a package of primary care, some inpatient care, and emergency care, as well as inpatient care at tertiary level public hospitals. Eventually, the government hopes to eliminate supply-side subsidies and provide uniform coverage for all.

Performance management, accountability and efficiency need to be improved to build on these gains.

Chile

Chile has statutory health insurance for workers, with no employer or government contribution. The health funds are managed by ISAPREs (Social Security Health Institutions).

The rest of the population is covered by a public fund manager, the National Health Fund (FONASA). These cover healthcare payments.

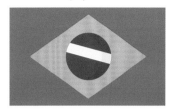

Brazil

Brazil has a government-run universal comprehensive public health system, funded by taxes at federal, state and municipality level. While the federal contribution is about 43% of total public health expenditure, municipalities contribute almost a third.

The system covers all types of healthcare for all citizens and visitors. However, wait times are unreasonably long at all stages, leading to out-of-pocket spending for basic care, while the delays push up treatment costs.

Drug unavailability leads to out-of-pocket spending. About a quarter of people have private health insurance, typically as an employment benefit.

National health expenditure is about 9% of the GDP. Most hospitals are public.

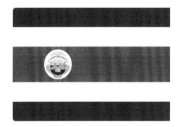

Costa Rica

Costa Rica also has a successful healthcare system, under a single-payer model that combines social security with the medical services offered by the Ministry of Health.

About 86% of the population has access to high-quality comprehensive care, which is delivered free. The rest are able to pay for care.

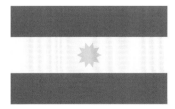

Argentina

Argentina has a healthcare system whereby insurance is provided and managed chiefly by workers' unions, while over a third of the population is uninsured and depends on public healthcare.

The good and the bad

South American healthcare systems suffer from poor resources, which are badly distributed to cover some areas. The capacity of the systems is low, and drug shortages are common. Corruption vitiates the process of official appointment and hampers reforms.

Response to COVID-19

The year of COVID-19 has seen over 21 million cases, and 560,000 deaths in South America, along with severe economic stress. Argentina, with a test positivity rate of 60 percent in October 2020 – the highest in the world - reflects both low testing and poor enforcement of non-pharmaceutical interventions.

Brazil has reported 13 million cases with over 330,000 deaths, with intensely divided political and public health messaging leading to it being one of the hardest-hit countries in the world. It is followed by Colombia, with a steadily increasing infection rate. Chile, meanwhile, has among the worst outbreaks in the world, with 1,500 deaths per million inhabitants.

The health response has been marked by its wide variation, with some countries instituting strict lockdowns, closing borders and eventually rolling out millions of vaccinations, while others have done almost nothing meaningful to prevent border crossing.

Limited resources, non-unified health systems, and poor social care, along with pre-existing unemployment and inequities, have led to a less than desirable response to the pandemic in most of Latin America, impacting the disadvantaged most severely, as expected.

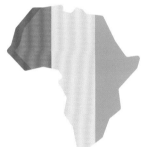

Healthcare systems in Africa

Sub-Saharan Africa has 13% of the world's population but carries a fourth of the world's disease burden. However, it spends only 1% of the global health expenditure.

Three out of four Africans have a per capita income of below $2 a day, and almost half spend less than $1 a day. Universal free healthcare is a right that is agreed to by all but is slow to become a reality.

Most Africans that are either low or middle-income turn to the public health system or to traditional healers. Only a few are able to afford high-quality private care, but nonetheless, out-of-pocket expenditures are bound to be high in this two-tier system.

Private spending accounts for 60% of all payments on healthcare. However, half of private healthcare expenditure is spent on private providers, and 40% of the lowest-income people in Africa pay for care from for-profit providers.

In Rwanda, national health insurance covers over 90% of the population, whereas less than 9% are covered in other countries.

Ghana has a National Health Insurance Scheme (NHIS), and built a public-private partnership network to reach areas without public health services. Funded through taxation, the NHIS covers most common diseases.

All residents must enroll and pay an annual premium, in return for free care. About a quarter lack any insurance, however. Almost 70% of those insured do not have to pay premiums, and underfunding challenges the working of the scheme.

In Kenya, a similar national health insurance program exists, for salaried employees, and for self-employed if they want to enroll. However, even this cost is inaccessible to most citizens.

So is the case with Tanzania, with its NHIF and CHF, for civil servants who pay 6% of their income, and for indigents and low-income people. In fact, most African countries share this situation, and national free healthcare accessible to those living in poverty is still a pipe dream.

Many countries spend only donor money on healthcare. Many times, international loans intended to improve the healthcare infrastructure had many strings attached. As a result, user fees were imposed on primary care. Drug pricing went up. Preventive and primary care was put out of reach of most low-income Africans.

Medicine became commercialized and privatized, and inequalities became more unequal. Infectious diseases like HIV emerged again. Government spending on health was cut due to required austerity measures.

Vacancies in the public sector increased, worsened by a freeze on recruitment and the flight of health professionals outside Africa. Most physicians went into private practice in urban areas, serving about 15% of the population. Drug shortages were endemic and intractable.

Cumbersome bureaucracy at all levels, inadequate coverage by insurance, low benefits for inpatient care, lack of transparency, and poor accountability, are the chief features of African health systems, in general.

This is worsened by the outflow of doctors to the US and other more lucrative and functional locations, and by ignoring the unique conditions of Africa in favor of western theories and policies. Poor sanitation and potable water facilities contribute greatly to this scenario.

Only six African countries spend 15% of their budgets on healthcare, and these are yet to achieve universal access to reasonable-quality healthcare.

COVID-19 response

African leaders showed solidarity in planning and executing interventions such as crossborder electronic cargo driver test result sharing, to prevent the spread of infections across countries. Lockdowns were implemented along with the closure of borders very early in the course of the spread of the pandemic to Africa.

Case finding, testing, contact tracing and isolation services were set up for free, as well as treatment. Public health education was enthusiastically provided to introduce proven non-pharmaceutical interventions such as masks, hand hygiene and social distancing.

Meanwhile, social support was put in place to support the economically weaker sections of society. Some waived fees on electricity and water and reduced house rents were announced in Ethiopia.

Advanced technology was used in Rwanda, including temperature-taking robots, drones for communication and surveillance, and pooled testing. Governmental transparency has been key to expert-driven decision-making, besides the unity displayed by political and health leaders.

Conclusion

Is there a perfect healthcare system? No, but the features that make for a good one include long-term investments in human resources and infrastructure, and in primary care (as in Israel). A Nordic focus on preventive care to improve population health and build capacity is important.

Public funding to allow the poorest to access healthcare and medication is an excellent model to follow, as in many Commonwealth and EU systems. Patient and community engagement, with an innovative streak, and a rapid response, is essential for maximizing coverage, like Rwanda and India.

Due investment in information technology and in research and development are key to making healthcare systems more accessible and improving health outcomes.

Lastly, attention to aged care, as in Japan, and to mental well-being, a mark of the Australian system, along with providing a choice of providers and services to the patient, seen in France, are fundamental to a healthcare system that follows best practices.

6 April 2021

References

Tikkanen, R. et al. (2021). U.S. Health Care from a Global Perspective, 2019: Higher Spending, Worse Outcomes? https://www.commonwealthfund. org/publications/issue-briefs/2020/jan/ushealth-   care-global-perspective-2019

Medical.mit.edu (2021). Healthcare in the United States: The top five things you need to know. https://medical.mit.edu/my-mit/internationals/healthcare-unitedstates

Healthmanagement.org. (2006). Facts & Figures: The UK Healthcare System. https://healthmanagement.org/c/it/issuearticle/facts-figures-the-uk-healthcaresystem

Great Britain: The National Health Service. https://sites.psu.edu/ smithcivicblog/2016/01/16/great-britain-the-national-healthservice/

Ec.europa.eu (2017). European semester thematic factsheet: Health systems.

Thorlby, R. (2021). International Health Care System Profiles England. https://www.commonwealthfund.org/international-health-policycenter/ countries/england

Earn, L. C. (2021). International Health Care System Profiles Singapore. https://www.commonwealthfund.org/international-health-policycenter/ countries/singapore

Gupta, I. (2021). International Health Care System Profiles India. https:// www.commonwealthfund.org/international-health-policycenter/ countries/singapore

World Health Organization. Regional Office for Europe, European Observatory on Health Systems and Policies, Miguel Á González Block, Hortensia Reyes Morales, Lucero Cahuana Hurtado. et al. (2020). Mexico: health system review. World Health Organization. Regional Office for Europe. https://apps.who.int/iris/handle/10665/334334

Kim, S. Universal Healthcare Systems and Fragmentation in Latin America. https://sites.google.com/macalester.edu/phla/key-concepts/ universal-healthcaresystems- and-fragmentation-in-latin-america

www.ilo.org. More than 140 million denied access to health care in Latin America and the Caribbean. https://www.ilo.org/global/about-theilo/ newsroom/news/WCMS_007961/lang--en/index.htm

www.un.org/africarenewal. December 2016–March 2017 | Vol. 30 No. 3

Fang, H. (2021). China. https://www.commonwealthfund.org/ international-healthpolicy- center/countries/china

Blumenthal, D. et al. (2020). Covid-19 — Implications for the Health Care System. The New England Journal of Medicine. https://www.nejm. org/doi/full/10.1056/nejmsb2021088

Apps.who.int. (2020). Mexico: health system review. https://apps.who. int/iris/handle/10665/334334

Altman, D. (2020). Understanding the US failure on coronavirus—an essay by Drew Altman. The BMJ. https://doi.org/10.1136/bmj.m3417. https://www.bmj.com/content/370/bmj.m3417

Scally, G. et al. (2020). The UK's public health response to covid-19. https:// doi.org/10.1136/bmj.m1932.   https://www.bmj.com/content/369/bmj. m1932

Ham, C. (2020). The challenges facing the NHS in England in 2021. https:// doi.org/10.1136/bmj.m4973.   https://www.bmj.com/content/371/bmj. m4973

www.thelancet.com. (2020). Building a resilient NHS, for COVID-19 and beyond. https://doi.org/10.1016/S0140-6736(20)32035-3. https://www. thelancet.com/journals/lancet/article/PIIS0140-6736(20)32035-   3/ fulltext

Han, E. et al. (2020). Lessons learnt from easing COVID-19 restrictions: an analysis of countries and regions in Asia Pacific and Europe. https:// doi.org/10.1016/S0140- 6736(20)32007-9. https://www.thelancet.com/ journals/lancet/article/PIIS0140- 6736(20)32007-9/fulltext

Child, J. et al (2020). Collaboration in crisis: Reflecting on Australia's COVID-19 response. https://www.mckinsey.com/industries/public-and-social-sector/ourinsights/ collaboration-in-crisis-reflecting-on-australias-covid-19-response#

Ihekweazu, C. et al. (2020). Africa's response to COVID-19. https://doi. org/10.1186/s12916-020-01622-w. https://bmcmedicine.biomedcentral. com/articles/10.1186/s12916-020-01622- w#citeas

Allin, S. et al. (2020). Comparing Policy Responses to COVID-19 among Countries in the Latin American and Caribbean (LAC) Region. https:// openknowledge.worldbank.org/handle/10986/35002

Gray, R. (2020). Lack of solidarity hampered Europe's coronavirus response, research finds. https://horizon-magazine.eu/article/lack-solidarity-hamperedeurope- s-coronavirus-response-research-finds. html

Macri, J. (2016). Australia's Health System: Some Issues and Challenges. Journal of Health & Medical Economics. https://health-medicaleconomics.   imedpub.com/australias-health-system-some-issuesand-challenges.php? aid=8344

Layland, A. et al. (2018). Are rankings the best way to determine healthcare systems?   https://healthmanagement.org/c/healthmanagement/ issuearticle/arerankings   the-best-way-to-determine-healthcare-systems

Jabukowski, E. et al. (1998). Public Health and Consumer Protection Series SACO 101 EN. Health care systems in the EU: A comparative study. https://www.europarl.europa.eu>saco>pdf

Zhai, S. et al. (2017). A study on the equality and benefit of China's national health care system. International Journal for Equity in Health. https://dx.doi.org/10.1186%2Fs12939-017-0653-4.   https://www.ncbi. nlm.nih.gov/pmc/articles/PMC5575878/

Azevedo, M. J. (2017). The State of Health System(s) in Africa: Challenges and Opportunities. In: Historical Perspectives on the State of Health and Health Systems in Africa, Volume II. African Histories and Modernities. Palgrave

Macmillan,   Cham.   https://doi.org/10.1007/978-3-319-32564-4_1. https://link.springer.com/chapter/10.1007/978-3-319-32564-4_1

'There is no quick solution to the nurse staffing crisis'

Government must be honest about nurse numbers and invest in the profession, says RCN, as new report shows significant shortfall of nursing staff in key areas.

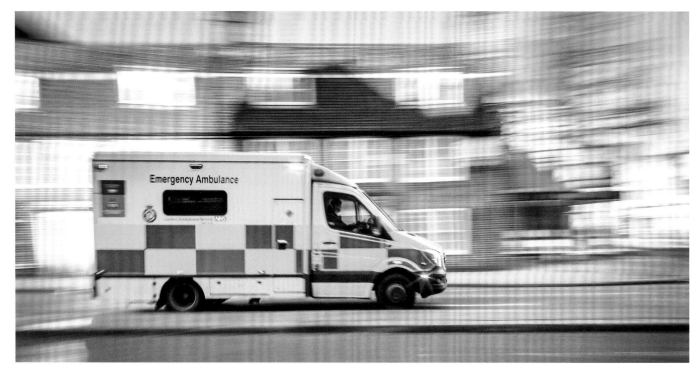

A report published by the Health Foundation today shows a decade of decline in the number of specialist mental health, community and learning disability nurses.

The report authors warn that nursing shortfalls, together with the backlog in routine care and growing need for health care, is likely to make recovering from the pandemic particularly challenging. They say the government will need to exceed its target of 50,000 new nurses in England by 2024/25 if it wants the NHS to fully recover from the pandemic.

The report shows that while overall nursing numbers have gone up by 8% since 2010, the number of health visitors and nurses working in community nursing, mental health and learning disability services are all lower than they were in June 2010.

The number of mental health nurses dropped by 8% in the 10 years to June 2020, health visitors dropped by 15%, there was a 12% drop in the number of community health nurses and a 39% fall in learning disability nurses.

The authors say the long-term trends are particularly concerning as people with learning disabilities are more vulnerable to COVID-19 than the general public, and the pandemic is likely to lead to increased demand for mental health services.

Responding to the findings, RCN Chief Executive & General Secretary Dame Donna Kinnair said: "This independent report paints a bleak picture, but it is one our nursing staff know all too well.

"There simply aren't enough to care safely for patients in hospitals, clinics, their own homes or anywhere else. The heavy demand on NHS and care services, long before the pandemic, was outstripping modest increases in staff numbers in some parts. The dramatic falls in key areas highlighted here, such as mental health, show we are getting further from what is needed – not closer.

"The report highlights concerning figures on the 'skill mix' too. Nursing support staff are a fantastic part of the nursing team but boosting their number should not come at the expense of investing in the registered workforce.

"There is no quick solution to this crisis. It will take honesty and investment on the part of government – paying people fairly for their skill and expertise and supporting the next generation of nursing staff through their education."

9 December 2020

Top 20 public health achievements of the 21st century

Public health has historically had a significant positive impact, improving the health and life course of the nation. As far back as 1848, the Public Health Act was instrumental in introducing sanitation, refuse systems and medical officers into local areas. In the last two centuries, we have seen major advances in medicine, hygiene, technology, planning, infrastructure, food, and many other areas that influence the public's health. This has resulted in the average life expectancy in the UK for a female born between 2016 and 2018 of 82.9 years.

But what has public health achieved more recently? Although we are generally much healthier than people were 150 years ago, there is still more to be done to tackle the modern health issues facing us. We compiled a long list of public health interventions and achievements that took place during the first twenty years of the 21 century in the UK. RSPH members voted, resulting in the shortlist which was ranked by senior public health professionals. These are the results.

1. The smoking ban

Probably the only entry on this list that almost any member of the public could tell you something about – and for good reason. The 2007 ban on smoking in enclosed public spaces was the kind of landmark legislation that just doesn't come around every year, marking a huge shift in the public mind-set. For most, the sight and smell of smoke-filled pubs, clubs, restaurants and workplaces are now a distant memory; for those too young to remember, it is probably hard to imagine that things were once this way at all. This speaks to the fact that, alongside the obvious health benefits of reduced smoking rates (both active and passive) since 2007, the indoor ban has been crucial in the denormalisation of smoking in public.

Perhaps most significantly, the smoking ban has helped shift the balance from the rights of smokers to poison others to the rights of others not to be poisoned. This has been reflected in the level of public support for the law, which has risen to 83% over the twelve years since its introduction. The ban is even backed by the majority of smokers nowadays – 52% of whom support it, with only 25% opposing. Polling by ASH earlier this year showed that popular support for Government to do more to limit smoking has increased leaps and bounds since the smoking ban, increasing from 29% in 2009, to 39% in 2017, and reaching 46% in 2019.

This shift has had wider consequences, arguably giving more oxygen to ideas that might once have seemed infeasible: smoking was banned in private cars with under 18s in 2015,

plain cigarette packaging was introduced in 2016, and we are seeing more and more local and voluntary initiatives for smoke-free public spaces outdoors. Just this year, the Government announced its ambition to end smoking by 2030, with a mandatory levy on industry as one option they will consider for funding this goal.

There is still much work to be done. Smoking remains the leading cause of preventable death and the picture for health inequalities is worrying – more must be done to bring down stubbornly high rates among routine and manual workers, and those with mental health conditions, for example. Nevertheless, the UK has made tremendous strides in bringing down rates, with the smoking ban underpinning and paving the way for the comprehensive programme of tobacco control that we see today.

2. The soft drinks industry levy ('sugar levy')

The Soft Drinks Industry Levy (SDIL) was introduced as part of the government's childhood obesity plan in April 2018. Manufacturers have to pay a charge for drinks containing over 8g of sugar. The levy has so far encouraged product reformulation, with the Public Health Minister reporting at the time of its launch that nearly half of the soft drinks market had been proactive in reducing sugar in their products to avoid charges. It also signalled a shift towards greater recognition of the role to be played by the food and drink industry in enabling healthier choices.

3. Marmot review into health inequalities and understanding of the social determinants of health

The Marmot Review of 2010 was a Government-commissioned report looking at the landscape of health inequalities in England, and what could be done about them. The review made a strongly evidenced case that health inequalities have social determinants, and that health and wellbeing were just as important measures for society as economic growth. While not being as well-known among the public as other entries to the ranking, the Marmot Review marked a real agenda shift for those working in public health. It reframed the narrative around determinants of health, and established a political imperative to tackle inequalities from a health perspective.

4. Sure Start children's centres (2000-2010)

Sure Start children's centres were designed to deliver a place in every community that would provide integrated care and services for young children and their families, with a particular focus on closing the achievement gap for children from disadvantaged backgrounds.

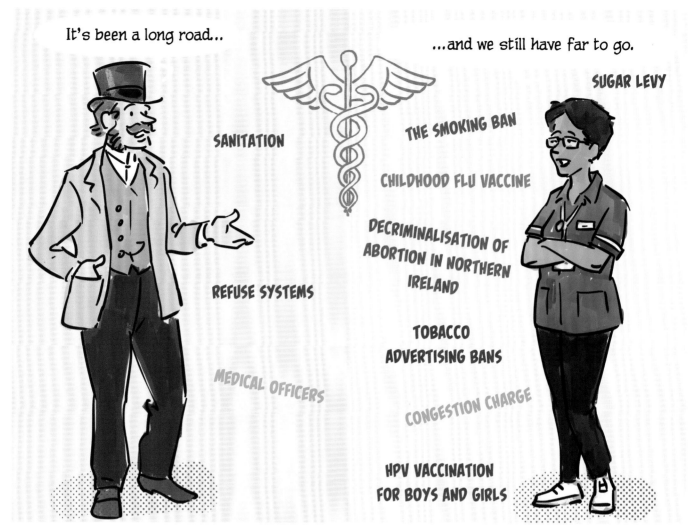

It's been a long road...

...and we still have far to go.

SANITATION

REFUSE SYSTEMS

MEDICAL OFFICERS

THE SMOKING BAN

CHILDHOOD FLU VACCINE

DECRIMINALISATION OF ABORTION IN NORTHERN IRELAND

TOBACCO ADVERTISING BANS

CONGESTION CHARGE

HPV VACCINATION FOR BOYS AND GIRLS

SUGAR LEVY

5. Minimum Unit Pricing on alcohol in Scotland

Minimum unit pricing (MUP) in Scotland for all alcoholic drinks was introduced in May 2018, following a string of court proceedings in which the Scotch Whisky Association fought against the legislation tooth and nail. The policy – which sets a minimum price of 50p under which a unit of alcohol cannot be sold – works by targeting the affordability of the cheapest alcohol products on the market, which is where the most harm sits.

Over the first year since implementation, MUP appears to have successfully reduced the amount of alcohol purchased by households in Scotland, with these reductions coming specifically within households that buy the most. Scottish ministers expect the changes to save almost 400 lives within the first five years of the new pricing rules. As a high profile example of a fiscal intervention that is effective in improving health outcomes, the policy has gained widespread support from many leading medical, public health, and police organisations. Wales, Northern Ireland and the Republic of Ireland are all at various stages of following Scotland's lead, and looking forward to the 2020s, it would be a great shame if England were to get left behind.

6. HPV vaccination for boys and girls

The introduction of a human papillomavirus (HPV) vaccine for girls aged 12-13 since 2008 has been a great success, with research in Scotland finding a dramatic reduction in cervical pre-cancer among vaccinated women. HPV also causes other cancers in both men and women. While most men are protected under a girls-only vaccination programme,

there are still many who are not, including men who have sex with men. To cover these gaps in herd immunity, the vaccine is now also offered to boys. Public Health England estimates that this universal programme will prevent 64,138 HPV-related cervical cancers and 49,649 other HPV-related cancers by 2058.

7. Congestion charge and ultra-low emission zone

The congestion charge was introduced in London in 2003, with the primary aim of cutting the number of private vehicles entering London during the day. It enforced a mandatory fee for vehicles driving within the Congestion Charge Zone (CCZ), and in 2019 this was taken a step further with the introduction of the ultra-low emission zone (ULEZ), coming into force across the same area as the CCZ. Both measures were brought in to tackle traffic rates by discouraging driving in this highly polluted area. Overall they have been successful interventions, with congestion reduced by 30% following the CCZ, and the ULEZ leading to substantial emissions reductions in NO2, CO2, and other pollutants.

Transport is a great example of a wider determinant of health. Though these two measures were primarily established for reasons only indirectly related to health outcomes, they have potentially huge ramifications in terms of road injuries, air quality, physical activity and mental health. As a result they have had a significant influence on the level of public debate around the relationship between transport, pollution, and our wellbeing.

8. Decriminalisation of abortion in Northern Ireland

Abortion in Northern Ireland was decriminalised in October 2019, allowing women and healthcare professionals to terminate a pregnancy without risk of prosecution. Up until this point, termination was only allowed if a woman's life was at risk or if there was serious risk of damage to her physical or mental health.

9. Wellbeing of Future Generations Act in Wales

In 2015 this act was brought in, requiring public bodies in Wales to think about the long-term impact of their decisions, to work better with people, communities and each other, and to prevent persistent problems such as poverty, health inequalities and climate change. Another example of the importance of legislation as a tool for improving public health, the Act is a momentous first step towards embedding the concept of inter-generational equity in everything we do, and changing health outcomes for the better for generations to come.

10. Tobacco advertising bans

There is a clear and extensive evidence base on the relationship between tobacco advertising and consumption, with children and young people being most susceptible to this influence. Historically, no one has been more aware of this link than the industry that has so successfully exploited it, driving forward the global tobacco epidemic by finding ever more inventive ways to market death in a stick.

Thankfully, in the 21st Century the UK has seen the steady but sure implementation of a comprehensive and wide-ranging set of advertising bans – starting with the Tobacco Advertising and Promotion Act of 2002. Beginning with a ban on print media and billboard advertising (2002), advertising and promotion of tobacco was subsequently banned at Formula One events through sponsorship (in 2002), at vending machines (in 2009), in point-of-sale displays in shops (in 2009), and finally through packaging (in 2016 – via the introduction of mandatory standardised 'plain packs').

11. Traffic light labelling on pre-packaged food

The traffic light labelling system was introduced by the government in 2013 as a clearer way to display nutritional information. The label includes information on calories, fat, saturated fat, salt and sugar. The system is currently voluntary, but there have been calls to make it mandatory due to the benefits for consumers.

12. Transferral of Public Health into Local Authorities

Responsibility for commissioning public health services was moved from the NHS to local authorities and the newly established Public Health England in 2013. At the time, the government ring-fenced a portion of public health funding for local authorities.

Despite being hamstrung by persistent cuts to the public health budget through the second decade of the century, councils have delivered improvements across 80% of the public health outcomes framework, and the rationale for local government leadership in public health remains sound. The strongest determinants of our health and wellbeing are the circumstances in which we live, and whether that means education, environment, housing or employment, local authorities remain well placed to influence these.

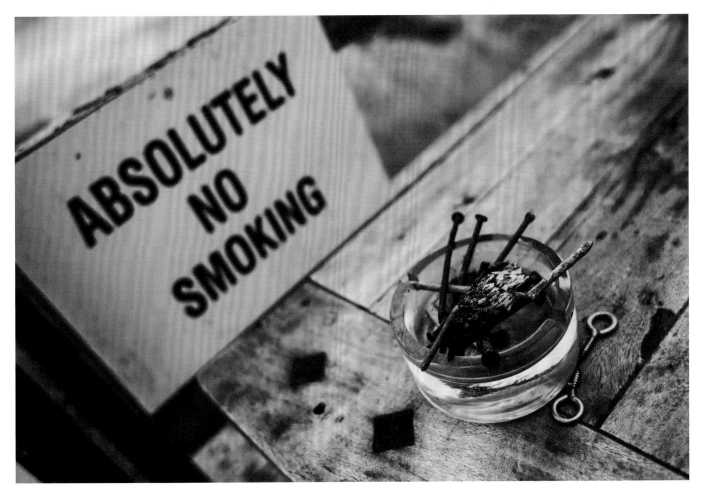

13. Scores on the Doors food hygiene ratings

Scores on the Doors started in 2005 as Food Hygiene Information collected by Local Authorities. The Food Standards Agency standardised the scheme, and in 2012 the Food Hygiene Rating Scheme was rolled out across every food business in the UK. Compliance across the UK has improved by 50% due to the initiative.

14. The Time to Change Campaign, run by Mind and Rethink Mental Illness

Time to Change is a campaign run by charities Mind and Rethink Mental Illness. It aims to improve public attitudes and behaviour towards people with mental health problems and reduce the amount of discrimination that people with mental health problems report in their personal relationships, social lives and at work.

15. Fixed-odds betting terminals stake limit reduced to £2

In 2018, the UK government reduced the maximum stake on Fixed Odds Betting Terminals (FOBTs) from £100 to £2. FOBTs have been described as the 'crack cocaine' of gambling, with their capacity to be played rapidly and repeatedly representing a serious addiction issue.

16. Introduction of childhood flu vaccine

The UK began primary-school-based pilots of child flu vaccination in 2013. They were a success, seeing falls in flu cases and influenza-related hospital visits for both children and adults in the community. Since 2019-20, flu vaccines are now rolled out for all primary school children in the UK every year.

17. Reduction in homelessness between 2003 and 2009

The 2002 Rough Sleepers Unit target to reduce the number of people sleeping rough by two-thirds was met a year earlier than planned. The recognition that rough sleeping was a product of a wide range of problems led to a new focus on prevention and recovery.

Following this, the Supporting People programme was launched in 2003 as a £1.8 billion ring-fenced grant to local authorities. Supporting People paid for accommodation-based services and interventions aimed at helping vulnerable people, including people who had been sleeping rough, to live independently.

The number of homeless households dropped sharply between 2003 and 2009 from 135,000 to just over 40,000. However, that number has since been rising steadily, up 50% between 2010 and 2017. Though this is still 56% below 2003 levels, homelessness remains a deeply ingrained and growing problem with strong ties to health inequalities – and it cannot be addressed without a sustained and well-funded commitment from the Government.

18. Junk food advertising ban during kids' TV and across London transport network

In April 2007, communications regulator Ofcom banned adverts for foods high in fat, salt and sugar during television programmes aimed at children under the age of 16, in an effort to curb childhood obesity. In February 2019, a similar ban across the Transport for London network came into force.

19. Drug safety testing at festivals and nightclubs

Drug safety testing is a harm reduction intervention that, especially in the second decade of the century, has been occurring in a growing number of countries worldwide – as well as notably in the UK, through extensive piloting at a number of festivals and nightclubs since 2013. It involves providing facilities where users can have their substances anonymously tested, after which they receive information on the strength and contents of the sample, along with tailored advice on how to minimise the harms from taking them. Drug safety testing pilots at two UK festivals in 2016 saw almost one in five users dispose of their drugs once aware of the content. When implemented at the Secret Garden Party festival in 2016, there was a 95% reduction in drug-related hospital admissions from the previous year.

The UK's spiralling drug-related deaths call for a far-reaching re-think of drugs policy, and safety testing can only be one part of the solution. However, it has been a totemic intervention within a growing movement towards a more compassionate approach to drugs policy – an approach that puts 'harm reduction' centre stage in pursuing a framework for reform that sees drug use first and foremost as a matter of public health, and not of criminal justice.

20. Cancer screening improvements

Bowel screening programmes began in England in 2006, Scotland in 2007, Wales in 2008 and in Northern Ireland in 2010. Patients aged 50 are offered a one-off bowel scope screening test. Research in 2017 suggested that bowel cancer incidence was 35% lower and mortality 40% lower among those screened. Breast cancer screening coverage also increased from 2002 to 2011.

Honourable mentions

Teenage Pregnancy Strategy for England

The English health inequalities strategy

Pre-exposure prophylaxis (PrEP) medication for preventing HIV

Introduction of Naloxone as an antidote for opioid overdoses

National Policy Planning Framework

These successes demonstrate the potential public health measures can have on improving health for all. We hope that the next twenty years of the 21st century continue to drive forward positive health outcomes, so that we all have the chance to live longer, healthier lives.

2019

Improving the nation's health through tackling obesity

By Stephen Colegrave

It's an uncomfortable truth: obesity is one of the biggest predictors for premature death in the UK today. It affects 35 million adults, and Nesta's Healthy Life Mission aims to halve its prevalence by 2030.

To investigate the opportunities and challenges, Nesta chief executive Ravi Gurumurthy chaired a roundtable gathering of health experts from across the food industry, the NHS, academia and the third sector. It brought together different perspectives on the problem, exploring how Nesta can help find solutions. The discussion was held under the Chatham House rule, and here's what we learned.

Understanding the issues around obesity

Nesta is approaching the obesity challenge primarily through the goal of improving food environments. That embraces physical factors like the availability of healthy, affordable options on our shelves and the influence of food advertising, but also people's individual circumstances – like their income or their ability to travel to shop. Taken together these elements can stifle people's freedom to make healthy choices, especially those living in areas of deprivation.

"We have to win public opinion on this issue. If you meet people where they are and tap into the existing motivations, you can engage people in the topic and take them on a journey."

To make sense of the challenge ahead, our panel first discussed the obstacles facing Nesta and our partners. We explored how the complex arguments that surround obesity are driving inertia. Our experts agreed there is a lack of understanding over the types of intervention that make the biggest difference – and an over-emphasis on changing individual behaviour and educating people to eat well. This can make it tough for individual players – retailers and manufacturers, political leaders and charities – to know how best to intervene. The panel felt that consistent messaging and practical support will be critical.

The fragmented food system is also an issue. Consumers buy from more than one source, so we need to examine the whole retail environment. Given that 96 per cent of retailers are small and medium-sized enterprises without the same knowledge and skill base as their larger competitors, our group felt a more nuanced, tailored approach is essential.

First off, it's important that everyone is moving in the same direction – and currently big players in the food industry are not in sync. Retailers and producers need to be convinced to work together, but competition laws currently bar them from doing so. It was noted, though, that those rules have been eased during the pandemic, and could feasibly be relaxed again. Conversely, the panel warned that good work

already being done by larger retailers is in danger of being undermined by discount stores, which are price-driven and historically harder to engage.

"The point about scale is that trying to get one solution that will work nationally across the board won't work for target communities, so a place-based focus is really important."

Participants felt we need to build on what has gone before, reframing and then scaling with the principles that have been tried and tested. Keeping the momentum going is key, and there's a need to scale up the many successful smaller initiatives – one speaker felt that focusing on one or two proven interventions would make that more effective. It was noted, though, that local contexts are vital: while some ideas could be rolled out at a national level, others will need more flexible, place-based approaches.

Next, attention turned to the stigma around obesity. It was generally acknowledged that weight is intrinsically linked with body image and mental health, sometimes fostering a fatalistic mindset on the issue – and this creates a challenge for our messaging. We need to confront the idea that tackling obesity is mostly about willpower. Participants agreed that weight reduction campaigns should include messages about body positivity to generate greater engagement.

We asked our roundtable guests which factors might prevent us from halving the prevalence of obesity by 2030, and they ranked their choices like this:

1. Public (mis)understanding of the causes of obesity
2. The tension between tackling obesity and promoting positive body image/mental health
3. The complexity of the issue
4. The fragmented food system
5. Insufficient data and evidence
6. Undefined roles of stakeholders
7. Maintaining momentum
8. Lack of clarity on best practice from industry
9. Balance of local/place-based vs national-scale interventions

It was agreed that public opinion needs to be won over, and that by meeting people where they live and tapping into their existing motivations, we can take them on a journey. But one speaker felt that it may prove difficult for individuals to translate our overarching messages into personal lifestyle changes.

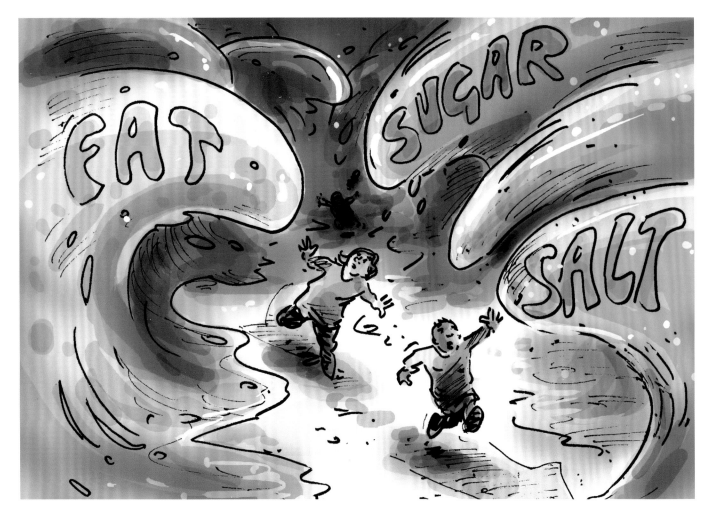

Regulatory regimes often set minimum standards that give little incentive for organisations to exceed them. Our panel discussed the levers we might pull to help companies recognise good practice and encourage investors and consumers to demand more. There is some willingness in the industry to take further steps, but this is hampered by a lack of clarity from government on how businesses could adapt.

Speakers also agreed that it's vital to consider deprivation and the related factors that influence individual food choices – factors like money, time and housing.

"None of these initiatives on their own are a silver bullet, it's going to need bringing them all together. You've got to lead on the things that the public is more prepared to run with."

Next steps for Nesta

Our group concluded that Nesta's best opportunity lies in directing attention to food environments, and starting with a local focus that benefits the maximum number of people, especially those from low-income backgrounds. They agreed it will be hard to make initiatives stick unless they're applied across all the food environments consumers interact with – that means looking beyond the major supermarkets to work with smaller retailers and fast-food outlets, baking in a bigger impact.

There was consensus, too, around capitalising on the momentum from recent policy measures, such as the sugar levy and the commitment to ban TV advertising of high fat, salt and sugar products before 9pm. Those changes demonstrate to the industry that more can and should be done. Nesta must interrogate the factors that will motivate businesses and investors to get on board, and encourage them to take action.

The panel also urged a reframing of the conversation. The issue of childhood obesity has won greater and more meaningful engagement by shifting the emphasis to focus on health, and a similar strategy could work for adults – perhaps by improving environments to support health rather than restricting personal choice.

Winning hearts and minds is vital, because at present there is a disconnect between the evidence and public attitudes to obesity. We need to explore ways to make people feel passionate about change in the food environment. Start with ideas they are more willing to sign up to, and we're more likely to achieve results.

We'd like to thank the participants who contributed to this roundtable. This is just the beginning of Nesta's journey into tackling obesity, and we'll continue to work with a range of experts and stakeholders as we proceed.

29 June 2021

UK in danger of failing a generation of children and young people, says new report

The RCPCH has published State of Child Health 2020, the largest ever compilation of data on the health of babies, children and young people across all four UK nations. The report shows that for many measures of children's health and wellbeing, progress has stalled, or is in reverse – something rarely seen in high income countries.

Across most indicators, health outcomes are worse for children who live in deprived areas. Inequalities in some outcomes have widened since the last State of Child Health report in 2017. Progress has also been seriously affected by deep cuts to local authority budgets - used to finance public health initiatives and community services.

The authors highlight that, even where there have been notable improvements in children's health, the UK is often lagging far behind other countries. For example, although there has been a fall in the number of emergency asthma admission rates across all four nations, the UK still has one of the highest mortality rates in Europe for children and young people with asthma.

Dr Ronny Cheung, Clinical Lead for RCPCH and co-author of the report, said:

Two weeks ago, the Marmot Review presented a stark picture about life expectancy in England. Now, our own report shows troubling signs for children and young people across the UK.

The harsh reality is that, in terms of health and wellbeing, children born in the UK are often worse off than those born in other comparably wealthy countries. This is especially true if the child is from a less well-off background.

Infant mortality is a globally-recognised sign of how well a country is looking after the health of its citizens. Throughout the world, the number of babies dying in their first year has been steadily falling for decades, as incomes rise and mothers and children receive better healthcare. Yet UK infant mortality rates have stalled, and in England they actually got worse between 2016 and 2017. For a high-income nation such as ours that should be a major wake up call.

State of Child Health 2020 brings together 28 measures of health outcomes, ranging from specific conditions – such as asthma, epilepsy, and mental health problems – to risk factors for poor health such as poverty, low rates of breastfeeding, and obesity.

Community paediatrician and co-author Dr Rakhee Shah, said:

Investment in preventative health services must now be prioritised by the new UK Government. England has seen a huge decline in spending on local services and I see the results of that every day of my working life especially for my most disadvantaged patients. The cuts to services also have an impact on our NHS – people have fewer places to go to get advice, support, and stay well.

The authors make a number of policy recommendations for each nation. For England, these include:

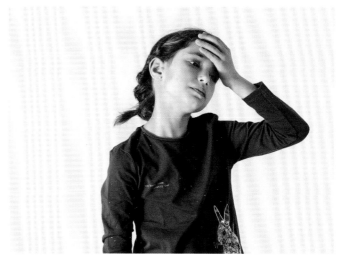

- Introduce a cross-departmental National Child Health and Wellbeing Strategy to address and monitor child poverty and health inequalities.

- Restore £1 billion of real-terms cuts to the public health grant for Local Authorities.

- Ensure future investment in public health provision increases at the same rate as NHS funding and is allocated based on population health needs.

- Implement in full commitments from the prevention green paper, Advancing our health: Prevention in the 2020s.

- Implement commitments to provide a Youth Investment Fund, with protection of the committed £500m funding.

- Provide health-based support for children throughout education, including funding for increased numbers of school nurses and school counsellors.

- Provide renewed investment in services for children and families, which support the child's school readiness.

- Ensure that health visiting services are protected, supported and expanded with clear and secure funding.

President of the RCPCH, Professor Russell Viner, said:

We've got a lot of work ahead of us if we're to get a grip on the state of child health in the UK. This report is the only one of its kind to zoom out and look at the full picture and it's not a pretty sight. On many vital measures we risk lagging behind other European countries.

There are some positive signs – teenage pregnancies have fallen hugely, Scotland is leading the way on reducing youth violence, and we've made huge strides in the treatment of conditions like diabetes. These outcomes are invariably the result of good policy, political commitment, and proper funding.

In many areas of healthcare, we've led the rest of the world. But we're in danger of failing a generation if we don't turn this situation around. The government has made welcome commitments on childhood obesity and young people's mental health but we need to see delivery in these and other areas. We have the evidence, the experience and the expertise to make real progress in the life of this government. It's now time to deliver for children and young people.

See below for some highlights of State of Child Health 2020.

Key highlights

Infant mortality

◆ The UK is fifth from bottom among 27 European countries for infant (under one year of age) mortality. Infant mortality in England stalled between 2013 and 2018 at 3.9 per 1,000 livebirths, with a slight rise in 2017 to 4.0.

◆ In England and Wales infant mortality is more than twice as high in the most deprived areas compared with the least deprived areas.

Healthy weight

◆ The prevalence of children aged 4-5 who are overweight or obese has not improved significantly in any of the four countries since 2006-7.

◆ Trends among 4-5 year olds are stable across the UK with around 25% of children overweight but this increases to around 34% for 10-11 year olds in England.

◆ Childhood obesity is more prevalent in deprived areas. In England, the prevalence of severe obesity among 4-5 year olds was almost four times as high in the most deprived areas (3.8%) than the least deprived areas (1.0%) in 2017/18.

Child poverty (new indicator)

◆ A total of 4.1 million children live in relative poverty in the UK (after considering housing costs) – an increase of 500,000 between 2011-12 and 2016-17. From 2016/17 to 2017/18, the numbers in England rose from 30% to 31% of children and in Wales from 28% to 29%

◆ Child poverty in Scotland plateaued at 24% and in NI decreased from 26% to 24%.

◆ Across the UK, rates of child poverty have increased for all types of working family. Lone parents working part time and households with only one working parent have seen the sharpest increases in poverty over the last three years.

◆ Nearly half of children (47%) in working lone parent families live in poverty.

Immunisations

◆ In 2018, all four UK nations fell short of the 95% WHO target for the second dose of MMR.

◆ In 2018, the uptake rates of two doses of MMR vaccine at 5 years ranged from 86.4% in England, 91.2% in Scotland to 91.8% in Northern Ireland and 92.2% in Wales.

Youth violence (new indicator)

◆ While rates of physical violence among young people are broadly similar across the four nations, England is the only country in which rates are increasing – most notably for 20-24 year olds. Between 2012 and 2017, the rate of physical violence among that age group increased from 297.7 to 315.49 per 100,000.

◆ In Wales, Scotland and Northern Ireland, physical violence among young people aged 10-24 shows an overall downward or stable trend from 2012-2017.

Long term conditions

Emergency admission rates for asthma have fallen since 2003/4 across the UK.

◆ However, the UK has among the highest mortality rates in Europe for children and young people with the underlying cause of asthma.

◆ Epilepsy had until recently seen similar falling rates of emergency admissions. However, in 2017/18 rates rose slightly in England, Wales and Scotland. In Scotland, children with epilepsy from the most deprived areas were twice as likely to have an emergency admission to hospital than those from the least deprived.

◆ There has been continued improvement in blood glucose control among children and young people with Type 1 diabetes across all four nations, and it is encouraging that there have been increases in the completion of key health checks for those with diabetes.

2020 indicators

◆ **Mortality** - Infant mortality; Child mortality (1-9 years); Young people's mortality (10-19 years)

◆ **Maternal and perinatal health** - Smoking during pregnancy; Breastfeeding

◆ **Prevention of ill health** - Immunisations / vaccinations; Healthy weight; Oral health

◆ **Injury prevention** - Accidental injury; Road traffic accidents; Youth violence (new indicator)

◆ **Healthy behaviours** - Smoking in young people; Alcohol and drug use in young people; Conceptions in young people

◆ **Mental health** - Prevalence of mental health (new indicator); Mental health services (new indicator); Suicide

◆ **Family and social environment** - Child poverty; Education – not in education, employment or training (NEET) (new indicator); Young carers (new indicator); Children in the child protection system; Looked After Children (new indicator)

◆ **Long term conditions** – Asthma; Epilepsy; Diabetes; Cancer; Disability and additional learning needs

◆ **Workforce** - Child health workforce (new indicator)

4 March 2020

www.rcpch.ac.uk

20 most common medical conditions affecting older people

By Josh

Around 26 million people in the UK have at least one long-term medical condition. This includes nearly 50% of people aged 65-74 and nearly two-thirds of those over 85. What's more, the UK's ageing population means these numbers will only increase in the coming years. In fact, experts predict that by 2030, around seven million older people will have at least one long-term illness or health problem. The ageing population and the increasing rates of long-term medical conditions have had a huge impact on the NHS.

Falls are a particular cause for concern. Even throughout the pandemic, falls remain the leading cause of emergency hospital admissions for older people. A fall can have a serious impact on long-term health, especially for those who suffer from a medical condition.

What is a medical condition?

'Medical condition' is a very broad term. It can refer to any kind of disease, disorder, injury, or illness, including mental illnesses. The older we get, the more likely we are to suffer from at least one medical condition. Some medical conditions are fairly mild and may not make much difference to your day-to-day life, while other medical conditions require intensive treatment.

But what are the most common medical conditions in the UK?

Common medical conditions in older people

Advances in healthcare have helped people in the UK live longer than ever before. As a result, medical conditions have become a more common feature of older life. Thankfully, there is more support than ever for people living with the most common health conditions.

It's important for us all to understand the most common medical conditions so that we are able to spot the symptoms and get medical assistance when we need it. Furthermore, we should understand how to prevent common illnesses and how to live with them.

Here's our guide to the most common medical conditions affecting older people.

1. Arthritis

Arthritis is one of the most common medical conditions among older people, affecting 10 million people in the UK. It causes joint pain and inflammation which can restrict your movement.

There are two common types of arthritis: osteoarthritis and rheumatoid arthritis. Among older people, osteoarthritis is more common. This is because osteoarthritis is caused by wear and tear; after all, the older we are, the more we have used our joints. Around eight million people in the UK have this type of arthritis. In contrast, rheumatoid arthritis is an autoimmune disease, where the immune system attacks the lining of the joints.

Symptoms of arthritis include:

- Joint pain, tenderness and stiffness.
- Restricted movement.
- Inflammation in and around the joints.

Unfortunately, there is currently no cure for arthritis. However, there are effective treatments such as painkillers and corticosteroids, which can help relieve the symptoms and slow down the condition's progress.

"Arthritis is a common condition that causes pain and inflammation in a joint. In the UK, around 10 million people have arthritis. It affects people of all ages. including children." – **NHS Choices**

The risk of a fall increases if you have arthritis. Therefore, people with medical conditions like arthritis (especially those who live alone) should ensure that they can always call for help if they need it. A personal alarm system lets you call for help 24/7. You simply need to push the red button on your pendant, worn around the wrist or neck, and our 24/7 Response Team will respond. For extra peace of mind, there is the Fall Detector alarm, which will call the Response Team automatically when it detects a fall.

A member of the team will assess your situation before taking the appropriate action. This usually means contacting your loved ones and informing them that you require urgent assistance. The team can also contact the emergency services when required.

2. Asthma

Asthma occurs when the body's airways are sensitive to allergens and become inflamed.

This inflammation can cause a painful and frightening asthma attack, which causes the airway muscles to tighten and narrow, making it hard to breathe. Most people can manage their asthma very effectively with proper medication. However, asthma left unchecked can be fatal. On average, 3 people die every day from an asthma attack in the UK.

Symptoms of asthma include:

- Coughing.
- A tight sensation in the chest.
- Breathlessness

Older people are susceptible to asthma and should be on the lookout for symptoms, especially during the winter months. Asthma can worsen during and after a bout of cold or flu.

Having a Personal Alarm could make a crucial difference if you suffer from an asthma attack. You can press your pendant button, which will instantly raise an alert with our

Response Team. They will communicate with you over the loudspeaker and arrange for help immediately. Should you collapse or fall while wearing a Fall Detector, your device will send an alert call automatically.

3. Blindness

Around two million people are living with sight loss here in the UK, with 360,000 people registered as blind or partially sighted.

The leading cause of blindness is age-related macular degeneration (AMD), which affects more than 600,000 people in the UK. AMD occurs when deposits build up on the macula (a small area at the centre of the retina). AMD can also be caused by abnormal blood vessels developing under the macula.

Other medical conditions can cause sight loss too – such as glaucoma and diabetes. Diabetic retinopathy damages the retina, leading to sight loss.

Treatments for sight loss vary depending on the cause, but may include:

◆ Cataract surgery.

◆ Eye drops.

◆ Laser surgery.

Early diagnosis of potential blindness is vital, so please seek medical attention if you notice any change to your vision. Of course, we should all have regular eye tests to ensure that our eyesight is healthy. The NHS recommends that people have an eye test every two years at the very least.

Sight loss can be very challenging to deal with. Luckily, there are several excellent support groups out there that can help – such as the RNIB.

4. Cancer

Did you know that 1 in 2 people will develop a form of cancer at some point in their lives?

There are over 200 types of cancer, such as breast cancer, prostate cancer and lung cancer.

Cancer is a disease where cells in the body replicate abnormally and form a mass known as a tumour. These abnormal cells multiply, either causing the tumour to grow or the cancerous cells to spread through the bloodstream.

◆ Here are some common cancer symptoms to look out for:

◆ Finding an unexpected lump.

◆ Unexplained weight loss.

◆ Unexplained blood in the stool, urine, when coughing, or when vomiting.

Smoking is one of the leading causes of cancer. If you are a smoker, there is no time like the present to quit smoking.

Thanks to medical research, cancer survival rates have been steadily improving for decades. Sadly, the survival rate is generally lower for older people. Therefore, it's very important to catch symptoms early and begin treatment as soon as possible. Please take a look at our guide to coping with cancer, an article we hope will help those affected by this condition.

5. Chronic Bronchitis

Chronic bronchitis is a condition that affects the lungs and airways. It's one of several lung conditions which come under the umbrella of COPD (chronic obstructive pulmonary disease).

Most cases of bronchitis develop as a result of an infection that irritates the bronchi (airways), causing an overproduction of mucus. The body tries to shift this excess mucus via coughing. Chronic bronchitis is when this coughing continues daily for several months of the year, for two years or more.

Look out for the common symptoms of chronic bronchitis, which include:

◆ Hacking cough, which may bring up mucus.

◆ A sore throat.

◆ Headaches.

◆ A runny or blocked nose.

◆ Fatigue.

◆ Aches and pains in your chest.

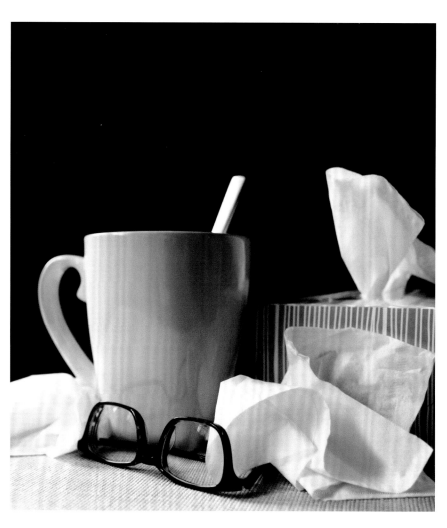

Smoking makes you more likely to develop chronic bronchitis and other COPD conditions. Therefore, the most important thing to do if diagnosed with chronic bronchitis is to quit smoking. Cigarettes will only make the condition worse and it will take longer to disappear. Alongside this, you should also ensure that you're eating a healthy diet to help prevent lung infections in the first place.

If you have chronic bronchitis, you should make sure that you get plenty of rest, drink plenty of fluids to avoid dehydration, and treat any headaches or fever with paracetamol or ibuprofen – but don't use the latter if you have asthma.

6. Chronic Kidney Disease

Chronic kidney disease (CKD) is quite common among older people here in the UK. There are several other medical conditions that affect the kidneys and can lead to chronic kidney disease. These conditions include kidney infections, high blood pressure, diabetes and kidney inflammation.

According to Kidney Care UK, around 64,000 people in the UK are receiving treatment for kidney failure – this is stage 5 chronic kidney disease, where kidney function is less than 15%.

Unfortunately, symptoms for the early stages of CKD are quite rare. In most cases, the condition is diagnosed during a blood or urine test for other medical conditions. As the condition progresses, you may suffer from:

- Shortness of breath.
- Feeling sick.
- Blood in your urine.
- Swollen ankles, feet or hands.
- Tiredness.

If you suffer from any of the symptoms above or notice any other worrying changes to your body, you should see your GP as soon as possible.

There is no cure for CKD right now, but there are treatments which can relieve the symptoms and prevent the condition from worsening. Options include medication, living a healthy lifestyle, dialysis or a kidney transplant in severe cases.

7. Coronary Heart Disease

Coronary heart disease is one of the leading causes of death here in the UK. According to the NHS, coronary heart disease (CHD) is what happens when fatty substances build up in the arteries, blocking the blood supply to the heart.

Certain lifestyle choices and other medical conditions can cause CHD. Risk factors include:

- Smoking.
- High cholesterol.
- High blood pressure.
- Diabetes.
- Obesity.

If you are at risk of CHD, your doctor might carry out an assessment. This could involve a treadmill test and one or more different scans. They'll also ask you questions about your family history and lifestyle. The main symptoms of coronary heart disease are angina, heart attacks and heart failure.

In order to reduce the risk of coronary heart disease, you might need to make important lifestyle changes. For example, everyone should take part in regular exercise and eat a balanced diet. Those who smoke should stop smoking as soon as possible. There are also several types of medication or surgery options to help treat CHD.

The knock-on effects of CHD can appear out of nowhere and can be fatal. If you have a Personal Alarm, you can raise the alarm as soon as you feel any chest pain, and help will be on its way within seconds. Remember, a Fall Detector Pendant will automatically detect a sudden fall and will automatically raise an alarm for you. Having this technology can make a huge difference should you suffer from a heart attack. We also offer a GPS alarm, which allows you to call for help both in your home and on the go.

8. Deep Vein Thrombosis

Deep vein thrombosis is a blood clot in your deep veins, most commonly in one of your legs. This medical condition is most common in people over the age of 40, and can also lead to further complications, including pulmonary embolism.

There are a number of factors that can increase your risk of DVT. These include obesity, blood vessel damage, being inactive for long periods of time, and a family history of blood blots.

In addition, smoking can cause serious damage to blood vessels. To lower your risk of deep vein thrombosis and several other medical conditions, you should seriously consider quitting.

Here are the most common symptoms of deep vein thrombosis:

- Pain, swelling and tenderness in one of your legs.
- A heavy ache in the affected area.
- Red skin – particularly at the back of your leg, below the knee.
- Warm skin in the area of the clot.
- A mild fever.

One common treatment involves blood-thinning medication, which makes it harder for the blood to clot and prevents existing clots from increasing in size. Alongside your medication, you will also need to make some lifestyle changes.

9. Dementia

Dementia is a progressive disorder that affects memory and overall brain function. It is relatively common in older people, affecting around 1 in 14 people over 65. This increases to 1 in 6 people over the age of 80.

The most common and well-known form of dementia is Alzheimer's disease. Vascular dementia is another type of dementia that develops as a result of a stroke or blood vessel deterioration.

Symptoms of dementia include:

- Difficulty remembering recent events.

- Problems in conversation – struggling to follow along or to find the right words.

- Difficulty judging distance.

- Forgetting where you are or what date it is.

Nearly one million people in the UK live with dementia, 90% of whom are 65 or over. If you notice any of the symptoms above, you should visit your GP as soon as possible, especially if you are over 65. An early diagnosis will help you get the best results from treatment while giving you more time to prepare for the future.

The symptoms of dementia can be frightening for you and your loved ones alike. Personal Alarms can offer peace of mind – especially the new GO GPS Alarm. If you ever get disoriented or become confused about your surroundings, you'll be able to press your pendant for help. Our expert Response Team are trained to provide reassurance and take action quickly.

10. Diabetes

Older people are susceptible to developing diabetes. In fact, half of all people with diabetes in the UK are over 65. Diabetes is a lifelong condition, which occurs when the body doesn't have enough insulin. This could be because the pancreas isn't producing enough, or because the body is resistant to the insulin it produces. Diabetes affects an astonishing 3.9 million people here in the United Kingdom.

Type 1 diabetes is an autoimmune condition, where the body attacks the cells that produce insulin. Type 2 diabetes, on the other hand, is when the body does not produce enough insulin or the insulin it makes doesn't work properly. This is the more common type of diabetes – affecting around 90% of diabetics.

Type 2 diabetes is a growing problem among older people, and a large proportion of newly diagnosed diabetics are from the older generation. In fact, one in 10 people over 40 are now living with this medical condition.

To help prevent type 2 diabetes, the NHS encourages the following lifestyle changes:

- Healthy eating – Increasing the amount of fibre in your diet and reducing sugar and fat intake.

- Maintaining a healthy weight – If you are carrying excess weight, lose it gradually by eating healthily and exercising frequently.

- Exercising regularly – It is important to stay active; perform both aerobic and muscle-strengthening activities.

11. Epilepsy

Epilepsy is a neurological condition that can cause seizures. Did you know epilepsy is most common in those at opposite ends of the age spectrum? It is most prevalent in young children and people aged over 65. In fact, 25% of people with epilepsy are over 65. Every day, 87 people are diagnosed with the condition.

Epilepsy can be caused by head injuries, strokes, tumours or certain infections. You'll normally receive a diagnosis if you've had two or more seizures. This is because many people have a one-off epileptic seizure during their lifetime.

There are several medications that can help to control epilepsy. In fact, these medications help eight out of every 10 people with epilepsy to control their seizures. If you have epilepsy, you should follow these steps to manage your condition:

- Stay Healthy – Take part in regular exercise and eat a balanced diet.

- Sleep – Ensure that you're getting enough sleep.

- Avoid Alcohol – Avoid excessive drinking.

Please remember that if you have a seizure and you currently hold a driving licence, you have a legal responsibility to inform the Driving and Vehicle Licence Authority.

A Fall Detector could be particularly useful to sufferers of epilepsy and similar medical conditions. This device will automatically raise an alert if it detects a fall. Our Response Team will then send help to your home immediately.

12. High Cholesterol

Cholesterol is a fatty substance that is created by your liver and is also found in some foods. Lipoproteins in the blood carry cholesterol around the body. There are two types of lipoproteins: low density and high density. You might have heard of "good" and "bad" cholesterol – "good" refers to high-density lipoproteins while "bad" refers to low-density lipoproteins.

High cholesterol is a medical condition that occurs when there is too much "bad" cholesterol in the body. A number of lifestyle choices and medical conditions can lead to high cholesterol. These include:

- Smoking.

- An unhealthy diet.

- Diabetes.

- High blood pressure.

- A family history of stroke or heart disease.

Age can also increase your chances of having high cholesterol, as the risk of your arteries narrowing is much higher. The best way to lower high cholesterol or prevent it in the first place is by living as healthily as possible.

This includes staying active by exercising or taking part in sporting activities, eating healthy foods, lowering your alcohol intake and trying to stop smoking.

13. Hypertension

Hypertension (high blood pressure) is one of the most common medical conditions in the UK. According to the NHS, more than one in four adults in the UK have high blood pressure. However, many people won't even realise it. The only way to find out is by having your blood pressure checked. Therefore, it's very important to have regular checkups with your GP, especially if you are in a high-risk group.

Noticeable symptoms of hypertension are rare. In fact, the only time someone will notice symptoms of hypertension is when their blood pressure reaches dangerously high levels.

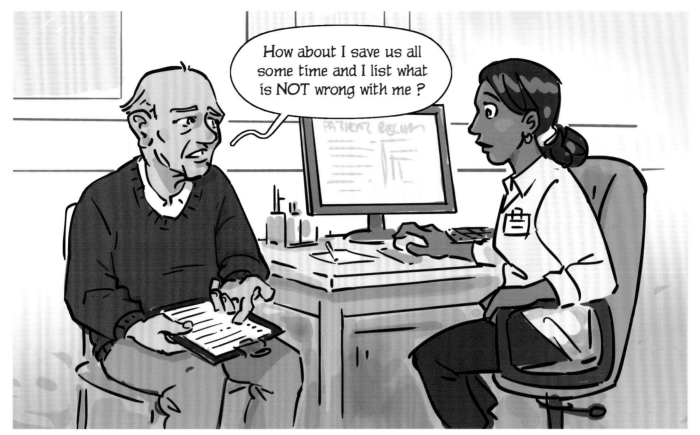

This is known as a hypertensive crisis. Symptoms of hypertensive crisis include severe headaches and anxiety, chest pain and an irregular heartbeat.

Hypertension puts significant strain on the blood vessels, heart, and other vital organs like the kidneys. As a result, people with high blood pressure are at higher risk of the following medical conditions:

- Heart disease.
- Heart attacks.
- Kidney disease.
- Vascular dementia.
- Strokes.
- Heart failure.

Here are some ways to prevent and manage high blood pressure:

- Watching your diet – Avoid foods high in saturated fat and sugar. Replace them with fruits and vegetables.
- Leading an active lifestyle – Begin adding more exercise to your day. Start by walking regularly and then move onto jogging if you can.
- Stop smoking – Nicotine raises your blood pressure and heart rate. If you smoke, quitting is the best decision you can make for your health.

The NHS recommends that all adults over 40 get their blood pressure checked at least every five years.

With a Personal Alarm, if you have chest pains or feel unwell, you can raise an instant alert by pressing your red button. Our Response Team will contact your loved ones and/or the ambulance service to come and assist you.

14. Motor Neurone Disease

Motor neurone disease is a rare neurological condition where the nervous system degenerates over time. It leads to muscle weakness and loss of mobility. Motor neurone disease, also known as ALS (Amyotrophic Lateral Sclerosis), occurs when the motor neurons that control activities like walking and speaking stop working.

Symptoms include:

- Difficulty swallowing (and sometimes excessive drooling).
- A weakened grip, usually in one hand at first.
- Small twitches and flickers of movement, known as fasciculations.
- Difficulty speaking or slurred speech, known as dysarthria.

The causes of motor neurone disease are still unknown. However, we do know that it affects more men than women and that it occurs most often in people between the ages of 50 and 70. Unfortunately, there is currently no cure for MND, but several treatments can minimise symptoms and slow the condition's progress. Despite being one of the rarer medical conditions on this list, it's relatively well-known, thanks to high-profile MND patients such as Stephen Hawking.

15. Multiple Sclerosis

Multiple sclerosis (MS) is a neurological condition that affects the brain and spinal cord. The main symptoms are a wide range of problems with vision, movement and balance.

There are currently more than 100,000 people in the UK living with the condition. The MS Society estimates that 5,000 more people are diagnosed with multiple sclerosis each year. That's approximately 14 people every day. This means that around one in every 600 people currently has multiple sclerosis.

Symptoms of MS include:

- Blurred vision.
- Muscle stiffness.
- Balance problems.
- Difficulty walking.
- Fatigue.

Currently, there is no cure for multiple sclerosis, although research into possible cures is ongoing. In the meantime, there are a number of treatments that can help to control the condition. Treatment options will depend on the individual's symptoms among other factors.

A personal alarm system can be a great reassurance for people with multiple sclerosis and their families. If you need help in an emergency, you need only press your Lifeline Alarm button. Our 24/7 Response Team will send help quickly, giving you the confidence you need to keep living independently.

16. Osteoporosis

Osteoporosis is one of the most common medical conditions affecting older people. More than three million people across the UK have osteoporosis, with more than 500,000 people receiving hospital treatment for fragility fractures every year as a result. This condition develops slowly over time and is often left undiagnosed until a fall causes a bone fracture.

This is because osteoporosis weakens the bones. Losing bone mass is a natural part of the ageing process, however, some people lose density faster than normal.

Women are more likely to have osteoporosis because they lose bone density rapidly after going through menopause. Luckily, certain medications can help to strengthen the bones.

Many people also take calcium and vitamin D supplements to maintain bone health.

According to the National Osteoporosis Foundation, certain exercises can help combat the condition:

Weight-bearing exercises – Activities that involve moving against gravity whilst staying upright. High-impact examples like skipping and tennis help to build bones and keep them strong. Low-impact examples such as using a stair machine or treadmill are safer alternatives for those who already have bone problems.

Muscle-strengthening exercises – Activities that involve moving the body, weights or other forms of resistance against gravity. Examples include lifting weights and using elastic exercise bands.

Osteoporosis and Falls

Falls are quite common among people with medical conditions like osteoporosis. Should you suffer from a fall, you may be unable to get back up or reach for your phone to call for assistance. Having a pendant button around your wrist or neck allows you to get help quickly after a fall. For added security, we would suggest the GPS Alarm, which includes built-in fall detection. This advanced device lets you call for help wherever you are.

17. Paget's Disease of Bone

Paget's disease of bone disrupts the normal cycle of bone renewal. It's triggered by a flaw in the bone cell regeneration system, which causes bone weakness and even bone deformity.

Paget's disease is a common bone condition that usually affects the pelvis, spine, and other areas of the body. It is a very common condition in the UK, mostly affecting people over the age of 50. The condition affects 8% of men and 5% of women by the age of 80.

Symptoms include the following:

- Constant, dull bone pain.
- Shooting pain that travels along the body.
- Numbness and tingling.
- Loss of movement in a part of the body.

These symptoms of Paget's disease can trigger a fall, which can be very dangerous if there is nobody around to help you. Having a Personal Alarm can help people who suffer from Paget's disease and other medical conditions. Simply press the red button on your pendant to call for assistance. Our Response Team will answer the call, assess your situation and arrange for help to come to you as quickly as possible.

18. Parkinson's Disease

Parkinson's disease is a chronic and progressive condition that damages certain parts of the brain. According to the NHS website, there are around 130,000 people in the UK living with Parkinson's disease. That's 1 in every 500 people.

The main cause of Parkinson's is a loss of nerve cells in a part of the brain called the substantia nigra. This leads to a reduction in dopamine, an important chemical in the brain. The condition is most common in middle-aged and elderly people.

The most common symptoms to look out for are:

- Involuntary shaking of particular parts of the body (tremor).
- Slow movement.
- Stiff and inflexible muscles.

Currently, there is no cure for Parkinson's disease. However, there are treatments available that can reduce the symptoms and help those affected to maintain their quality of life for as long as possible.

19. Stroke

Having a stroke can be life-threatening if you don't seek medical attention straight away.

A stroke occurs when the blood supply to a part of your brain is cut off. Without blood, brain cells can be damaged and may even die.

Strokes are particularly common among older people. The average age for suffering a stroke is 74 for men in England, Wales and Northern Ireland. For women, however, the average age is slightly higher – 80. Across the UK, strokes are a leading cause of disability, with around two thirds of all survivors being left with a disability of some kind.

It's very important to know the signs and symptoms of a stroke. The sooner you get treatment, the better the outcome is likely to be. As mentioned, strokes can be life-threatening, so it's important to seek medical help as soon as possible. Memorise the signs of a stroke with the word FAST:

Face – Has their face drooped or fallen on one side? Can they smile?

Arms – Can the person raise both arms and hold them there?

Speech – Are they speaking clearly? Or is their speech slurred or garbled?

Time – Don't waste any time! Dial 999 immediately if you notice any of these symptoms.

It's absolutely vital to call 999 if you notice any signs of a stroke. Wearing an alarm pendant ensures that you can call for help even if there's no one around or you're unable to reach for the phone. Our Response Team will take care of everything, by calling the emergency services and notifying your loved ones. They'll also be able to inform the paramedics of any other medical conditions you have, as well as any allergies and medications you take.

20. Shingles

Shingles is a skin condition that is very common among older people, especially those over the age of 70. This is because your body's immune system becomes weaker as you age.

Shingles is caused by the same virus which causes chickenpox. Therefore, only those who have had chickenpox can develop shingles. The infection will usually cause a painful rash and/or blisters to form on your skin, which may become extremely itchy.

If you have shingles, the affected area will feel quite tender and you may experience sharp stabbing pains every now and then. Other symptoms include a burning and tingling feeling in the affected areas, as well as a high temperature and a general feeling of being unwell.

The sooner you see a doctor, the sooner treatment can begin. The NHS suggests using calamine lotion as this has a cooling, soothing effect on the skin and can relieve the itchy feeling. If your blisters are weeping, you can use a cloth or flannel which has been cooled with tap water to relieve discomfort.

People aged 70-78 are eligible for a free shingles vaccination with the NHS. This is the best way of avoiding the condition.

19 July 2021

Alarming new data shows the UK was 'sick man' of Europe even before Covid

A global study has exposed how poorly prepared Britain was for a virus that targets our most vulnerable people.

By Richard Horton

Our health is determined by far more than a single virus. This week, a team of scientists in Seattle, together with thousands of contributors around the world, assembled 3.5bn pieces of data to construct what they are calling the Global Burden of Disease. The story this data tells us about Britain is alarming. On some of the most important measures of health, the four nations of the United Kingdom perform worse than our nearest neighbours. Even with coronavirus out of the picture, Britain is the sick man, woman and child of Europe.

The headline findings from the report are clear. In 2019, life expectancy at birth in the UK was 82.9 years for a woman and 79.2 years for a man (the average for both was 81.1 years). These numbers look good, especially when compared with historical figures. In 1950, for example, the average life expectancy at birth for a UK citizen was 68.9 years. The combined effects of economic growth, better education and an improved NHS have delivered an extra 12 years of life. Impressive.

That is until you start comparing the UK with other European countries. When you do this, you find we have seen smaller increases in life expectancy than the western European average. Spain and Italy, for example, both had an average life expectancy at birth of 83.1 years in 2019. In France, it was 82.9 years, Sweden 82.8 years and Germany 81.2. The western European average life expectancy was a whole one year longer than in the UK.

Another important measure is what's known as healthy life expectancy – the years of life we spend in good health. The average healthy life expectancy for the UK in 2019 was 68.9 years, meaning that people in the UK spend an average 12.2 years living with some kind of illness. And again, when one compares the UK with other European nations, we perform poorly.

In fact, Britain has the worst healthy life expectancy of any other European country. We come bottom of the league table, alongside Monaco. We've seen a slower improvement

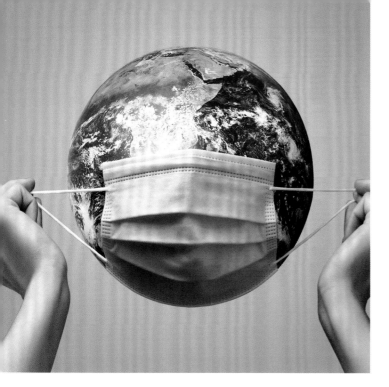

in healthy life expectancy (3.6 years) than the western European average (5.8 years). And the situation for children is equally bad: the under-five mortality rate in the UK in 2019 was 4.1 deaths per 1,000 live births – one of the worst performances in western Europe, second only to Malta. Whatever metric one chooses, the UK's health performs worse than comparable European nations.

There's a similar pattern at play across the four nations. Scotland has the lowest life expectancy (79.1 years), followed by Northern Ireland (80.3 years), Wales (80.5 years), and England (81.4 years). What's going on?

The major causes of Britain's poor health are noncommunicable diseases such as diabetes, chronic respiratory disease and dementia. The Global Burden of Disease shows that deaths from alcohol and drug use have increased by 280% and 166% respectively over the past 30 years. And the health of our nation is not uniform across the country. There's an eight-year difference in life expectancy between the north and the south of the UK. Life expectancy is highest in Richmond (84.5 years) and lowest in Blackpool (76.4 years) – worse than the average for China, Turkey, Thailand, Cuba, Chile, Jordan and even the US.

These differences in life expectancy hold a mirror up to the inequalities across our nation.

The lowest 10 expectancies in England skew towards the poorest places in the north-west and north-east of the country: Blackpool, Middlesbrough, Hull, Liverpool, Hartlepool, Rochdale, St Helens, Sunderland, Blackburn and Manchester. And here one finds an interesting and important correlation. Is it a coincidence that the worst life expectancies in England track the upsurge in coronavirus? I don't think so.

The pandemic is not the making of a single coronavirus, but the combination of three epidemics: the virus, the chronic conditions that make people more susceptible to it, and a situation of deepening poverty and inequality. A single pandemic is too simple a narrative to capture this reality. What we're faced with in Britain is a "syndemic" – a synthesis of epidemics.

The reasons we have been so devastated by this virus are reflected in the Global Burden of Disease in 2019, which exposes how poorly Britain was prepared for a virus that targets the least healthy in our society. Overcoming this crisis will involve far more than just preventing transmission. To protect our communities from coronavirus we will need to address the underlying diseases that leave people vulnerable, and the inequalities that scar our society.

This government has so far failed to offer an adequate strategy for either. Take obesity as an example. After Boris Johnson contracted coronavirus, he promised to make tacking this condition a priority, conceding that "losing weight, frankly, is one of the ways you can reduce your own risk from coronavirus". But the government has so far left the root causes of obesity – the junk food industry, the difficulty of accessing affordable healthy produce, and the fact that many people in poverty lack the time to prepare food from scratch – untouched.

The virus has exposed the inequalities that divide our society. It is deprived areas such as Bolton and Rochdale where infections have been endemic. It's no accident that Liverpool, which scores high on the list of the UK's most deprived places, was the first region to be classified as very high risk in Johnson's recalibrated approach to Covid-19.

Yet the government remains silent on a plan for reversing or reducing these disparities that have left our citizens so unprotected. Beyond empty platitudes and promises to "level up" the country, Johnson rarely if ever talks about inequality. And when he does, Johnson frames the subject in positive terms; in 2013, he famously quipped that "some measure of inequality is essential for the spirit of envy and keeping up with the Joneses that is, like greed, a valuable spur to economic activity". It's this tolerance for inequality that explains why Britain has such gaping disparities in life expectancy between rich and poor areas, and why the virus has hurt those latter places so badly.

At the beginning of the pandemic, 1.5 million people in England were deemed at sufficiently high risk of coronavirus to require shielding. The unfortunate truth is that far more people in the UK are at risk than this number suggests. As work from University College London revealed earlier this year, when one includes those over 70 years of age, and those who are under 70 but live with chronic diseases such as diabetes or cancer, the actual number at risk in the UK is more than 8 million people.

This pervasive political indifference to inequality, combined with a decade of cuts to the most basic social protections, has left our nation exquisitely vulnerable to the arrival of this virus. A national revival is possible. But only if our government takes the health of its citizens seriously. The signs so far are that it does not.

18 October 2020

Richard Horton is a doctor and edits the Lancet

Health of 12 million Brits at risk from climate crisis

More than 12 million people living in the UK are vulnerable to the physical, mental and health impacts of the climate crisis, a new report has warned.

By Matt Mace

A new report from The Climate Coalition and the Priestley International Centre for Climate has warned that the health of more than 12 million people could deteriorate as heatwaves and major flood events rise in frequency and impact as a result of the climate crisis.

Approximately 1.8 million people in the UK are living in areas that are at significant risk of flooding, according to the report, a number that could reach 2.6 million over the next 17 years. The report notes that flooding can worsen mental health and wellbeing, with one third of people that have experienced flooding also experiencing Post Traumatic Stress Disorder (PTSD).

Additionally, around 12 million people – namely the elderly and those with pre-existing health conditions - are vulnerable to the impacts of heatwaves.

In the UK, heat-related mortality in people older than 65 years increased by 21% between 2004 and 2018, the report notes. In 2020, 16 nights were recorded where the temperature remained above 20C and heat-related deaths reached 8,500 in 2018.

The report from the Climate Coalition, whose members include National Trust, WWF, Women's Institute, Oxfam and RSPB, therefore calls on the UK to play its part in tackling the climate crisis. Doing so would improve air quality and reduce the pressures being place on the NHS.

The Climate Coalition's campaigns director Clara Goldsmith said: "Failure with speed and scale to address the climate and ecological crises will spell disaster not only for our natural world, but for public health. Governments must urgently recognise the threat posed by climate change and set the recovery on a green pathway that enshrines planetary and public health above all else."

According to WWF, rising sea levels, storms and flooding driven by climate change has placed more than £12bn of the UK's economy at risk, while almost 2.5 million homes in the UK could suffer from flooding by 2050.

Coastal protection is largely provided by saltmarshes and seagrass beds. Yet the UK has already lost up to 92% of its seagrass in the last century and 85% of its saltmarsh. WWF's chief executive Tanya Steele added: "Our mental and physical health are clearly linked to the health of the one place we all call home: our planet. Yet right now, nature - our life support system - is in freefall, and the climate crisis is making blazing heatwaves and major flood events more frequent and more likely.

"To show true global leadership at this year's climate summit, the UK Government must take more ambitious

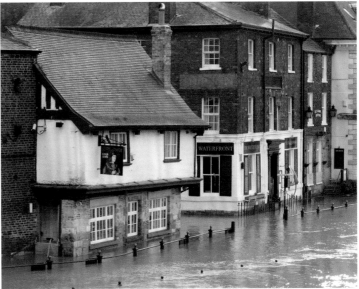

steps to reach our net-zero targets and put nature on the path to recovery."

Business resiliency

There are business risks to consider too. Indeed, it is estimated that flooding damage cost UK businesses £513m in 2015 alone.

A survey of 122 of the UK's biggest businesses found that half have done little or no work to prepare for climate change risks - both physical and transition-related. The survey was conducted by the Chartered Institute of Internal Auditors (Chartered IIA) and The Climate Group. It polled chief audit executives at 67 FTSE-100 firms and 55 other large businesses on their approach to preparing for climate change.

While more than two-thirds of the respondents said climate change will present risk to their business in the short to medium-term, 52% revealed that they have done either little or no work so far to prevent climate-related risks.

Separate research from Cervest found that three-quarters of UK businesses are concerned about climate-related risks, just one in ten consider measuring and disclosing their climate-related risks a priority.

5 February 2021

Nuffield research shows 8.8m Brits have done no exercise in the last 12 months

By Tom Walker

- **A new study from Nuffield has highlighted the impact of lockdown on exercise habits**
- **8.8m have done no exercise in the last year**
- **73 per cent of Brits are failing to meet NHS exercise guidelines**
- **A third say their physical health is worse than it was a year ago**

Nearly three in four (73 per cent) Britons are failing to meet NHS recommendations on exercise, as a result of successive lockdowns leading to the formation of unhealthy habits.

In addition, there's evidence of a growing mental health crisis, as 41 per cent of Brits say their mental health has become worse in the past year.

The figures come from The Nuffield Health Healthier Nation Index, launched by the healthcare charity, which is based on a comprehensive survey of more than 8,000 Britons.

Nuffield says the study offers one of the most detailed looks at the nation's health since the start of the pandemic.

The Index reveals that, on average, a third of Britons (33 per cent) agree their physical health is worse now (April 2021) than it was a year ago, with older age groups reporting a worse decline.

Strikingly, only 10 per cent of those over 55 years of age agreed their physical health has improved.

Despite well-publicised evidence pointing to the link between obesity and severity of illness from COVID-19, and in the wake of the Prime Minister announcing a new obesity strategy last year, 16 per cent of the population – which accounts for an estimated 8.8 million adults – have done no exercise at all in the last 12 months.

This rises to a quarter of over 55s, despite research showing a lack of exercise to be one of the highest risk factors for death from COVID-19.

Reflecting on the findings, Judy Murray OBE, ambassador for the The Nuffield Health Healthier Nation Index, said: "This research shows that the pandemic has had a significant impact not only on the nation's mental health – but also on our ability to exercise.

"The focus must now be on helping people get active to make sure we don't store up problems for the future.

"It is deeply worrying that 1 in 4 people over the age of 55 haven't exercised at all in the last year.

"We need to make sure everyone has the tools they need to look after their mental and physical health, and everyone should see 2021 as a critical opportunity to prioritise their health and wellbeing."

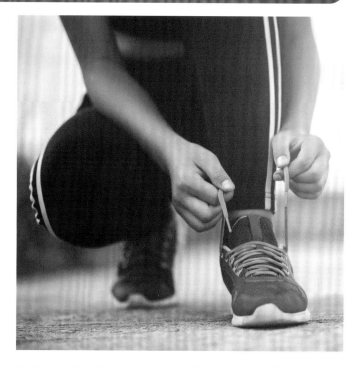

Dr Davina Deniszczyc, Medical Director at Nuffield Health, said: "The findings from the Healthier Nation Index show the stark effect COVID-19 is having on people's physical and mental health. There are some worrying trends that if not addressed could see us sleepwalking into another type of health pandemic.

"It is essential that we now focus on national recovery and the prevention of long-term health conditions such as obesity, diabetes and heart conditions.

"It's shocking to see the levels of inactivity with the vast majority of people failing to meet NHS guidelines for exercise and many older people haven't been doing any exercise at all.

"We need to do everything we can to increase exercise rates, reduce long term health conditions if we are to build the resilience of the nation's health and avoid another health crisis."

20 May 2021

What next for the future of health security in the UK?

The Mental Health Foundation responds to today's proposals for the new UK Health Security Agency.

By Antonis Kousoulis, Director of England and Wales

Whatever the intent, the proposal announced today for the future of Health Security in England will result in a more fragmented system. We are losing a single national public health body (Public Health England) that currently provides a clear, integrated and cohesive focus on health improvement, and, within this, public mental health.

While the new UK Health Security Agency has a broad public health remit, its predominant focus is on infectious disease control, not creating the conditions and supporting the action needed in our communities to enable people to enjoy good overall health.

It is, of course, vital that the UK is in a good position to respond to pandemic threats. However, in public health terms, health security is a holistic term: the protection from threats to our health. Considering that not all pandemics can be prevented, it is also vital, then, that the country is able to respond effectively to the threats that pandemics pose to the overall health of our country's citizens and the fabric of our society, including their mental health. Health security is understood in both a collective way – reducing the vulnerability of communities to harms to health – and an individual way – access to safe and effective products, services and technologies.

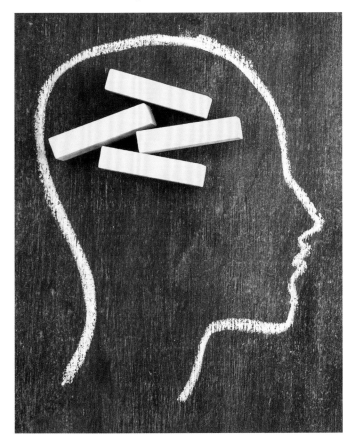

If this past year has taught us anything, it is that an effective response to pandemics also means holistically addressing the risks to people's mental health, supporting those who are most vulnerable, and tackling those persistent inequalities that cause many communities to have very different health experiences to others.

The devastating loss of life, months of social isolation and widespread financial instability we have seen over the last year because of Covid-19 has brought despair to individuals, families and communities. Before the crisis, many people in our society with mental health problems were already struggling to access the basic support needed to stay well.

With hundreds of thousands more people likely to experience mental health problems as a result of the pandemic, continuing with business as usual is now not an option. The creation of this new agency – the announcement of which contains no reference to the mental health effects of the infectious disease pandemics – is far from being the whole of the change we need to see.

People's experiences during this time do not have to lead to mental health problems in the future if we have a comprehensive plan to deal with the aftermath of the pandemic. In addition to the human cost of mental ill-health, there are compelling economic reasons to ensure that, as we return to living our lives as we used to, we are all able to thrive and play a full part in the national recovery. We are still awaiting the Government's cross-government mental health recovery plan and would like to see this published as soon as possible. The Government needs to be clear what its ambitions are, how they will be measured, and who will be held to account for their delivery.

The Government has today signalled that it will soon be publishing its proposals for the future of national health promotion and health improvement functions, and we will be scrutinising these carefully to see what they mean for public mental health. It is vital that all parts of the new system are fully accountable for working well together and that public mental health remains a strategic and cross-cutting priority, as it currently is for Public Health England.

24 March 2021

- The National Health Service was formally founded in 1948. The passing of the National Health Service Act for England and Wales was overseen by Aneurin 'Nye' Bevan. (page 1)

- In 2018/19 the UK spent around £153bn on health, in 2019/20 prices. This is an increase of 2% compared to the previous year and is ten times more than was spent sixty years earlier, in 1958/59. (page3)

- On average health spending has increased by 3.6% a year over the history of the NHS as a result of the UK's growing population, the increasing prevalence of chronic conditions, and the rising costs of delivering care. (page 3)

- Over the last decade, growth in health spending has slowed, reaching just 1.6% a year since 2011/12. At that point health spending was 7.3% of GDP, a drop since its highest level of 7.6% in 2009/10. (page 3)

- Polling by Ipsos MORI, conducted ahead of a webinar co-hosted with the Health Foundation, shows that three-quarters of British adults say that Britain's NHS is one of the best in the world. (page 4)

- The number of beds in English NHS hospitals has halved in the last 30 years (from 299,000 in 1987-88 to 141,000 in 2018-19). Likewise, the UK has 2.8 doctors per 1,000 population compared to 4.0 in Italy or 4.3 in Germany. (page 6)

- More than half of trainee doctors (56 per cent) working for the NHS are considering only working part-time hours, according to figures released by a royal college. (page 7)

- A poll of 2,019 adults commissioned by Healthwatch found 61% of respondents felt that NHS dental treatments were expensive. (page 11)

- People living in the North East of England are the most likely to avoid NHS dental treatment due to costs (13%), compared with just one in 30 (3%) who live in the South West. Despite this, people in the North East have been charged for NHS dental treatments the most (29%), while people in the South West were charged the least (13%). (page 12)

- The National Health Service (NHS) is 79% publicly financed from taxes, and operated by the Department of Health. About 20% is paid for by national insurance, and private patients and co-payments make up the rest. (page 13)

- The number of NHS mental health nurses dropped by 8% in the 10 years to June 2020, health visitors dropped by 15%, there was a 12% drop in the number of community health nurses and a 39% fall in learning disability nurses. (page 20)

- As far back as 1848, the Public Health Act was instrumental in introducing sanitation, refuse systems and medical officers into local areas. (page 21)

- The indoor smoking ban was introduced in 2007 in the UK. (page 21)

- The HPV vaccine has been routinely offered to all girls aged 12-13 in Britain since 2008. (page 22)

- The UK began primary-school-based pilots of child flu vaccination in 2013. They were a success, seeing falls in flu cases and influenza-related hospital visits for both children and adults in the community. Since 2019-20, flu vaccines are now rolled out for all primary school children in the UK every year. (page 24)

- Obesity is one of the biggest predictors for premature death in the UK today. It affects 35 million adults. (page 25)

- Around 26 million people in the UK have at least one long-term medical condition. This includes nearly 50% of people aged 65-74 and nearly two-thirds of those over 85. (page 29)

- 1 in 2 people will develop a form of cancer at some point in their lives. (page 30)

- There are over 200 types of cancer, such as breast cancer, prostate cancer and lung cancer. (page 30)

- Diabetes affects 3.9 million people in the United Kingdom. (page 32)

- The average age for suffering a stroke is 74 for men in England, Wales and Northern Ireland. For women, however, the average age is slightly higher – 80. (page 34)

- Nearly three in four (73 per cent) Britons are failing to meet NHS recommendations on exercise, as a result of successive lockdowns leading to the formation of unhealthy habits. In addition, 41 per cent of Brits say their mental health has become worse in the past year. (page 38)

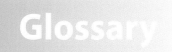

Coronavirus/COVID-19

Coronaviruses are a large family of viruses that cause respiratory infections. These can range from the common cold to more serious diseases.

COVID-19 is caused by a new form of coronavirus known as SARS-CoV-2 (severe acute respiratory syndrome coronavirus 2). It was first reported in December 2019.

Herd immunity

Herd immunity is the indirect protection from a contagious infectious disease that happens when a population is immune either through vaccination or immunity developed through previous infection.

Immunisation

A process by which a person becomes protected against a disease through vaccination. This term is often used interchangeably with vaccination or inoculation.

Lockdown

A lockdown is a restriction policy for people or community to stay where they are for health and safety reasons. For example: limiting travel, social interaction and access to public spaces to mitigate the spread of a contagious disease like COVID -19.

National Health Service Act

The National Health Service Act came into effect on 5 July 1948. The Act provided for the establishment of a comprehensive health service for England and Wales. There was separate legislation produced for Scotland and Northern Ireland. The first Minister of Health was Aneurin Bevan MP.

NHS

NHS stands for National Health Service. It refers to the Government-funded medical and health-care services that everyone living in the UK can use without being asked to pay the full cost of the service.

Pandemic

A pandemic is a disease outbreak that spreads across countries or continents. It affects more people and takes more lives than an epidemic. The World Health Organization (WHO) declared COVID-19 to be a pandemic when it became clear that the illness was severe and that it was spreading quickly across the globe.

PPE

PPE stands for Personal Protective Equipment. PPE is designed to protect you from harmful substances such as chemicals or infectious agents. In a pandemic situation, it can also help prevent the transmission of infection between staff and patients.

Public Health Act 1848

The 1848 Public Health Act was established to improve public health via the introduction of sanitation, refuse collection systems, the provision of clean drinking water and the appointment of a medical officer for each town.

Stroke

A stroke is a medical emergency. It occurs when the blood supply to part of your brain is interrupted or reduced, preventing brain tissue from getting oxygen and nutrients. Brain cells begin to die in minutes.

Vaccination

Vaccination is the act of introducing a vaccine into the body to produce immunity to a specific disease.

Activities

Brainstorming

◆ Brainstorm what you know about the NHS and the health issues in the UK.

- What is the NHS?

- When and why was the NHS set up?

- What are the biggest problems facing the NHS today?

- What do you think is the biggest health issue for people in the UK today?

- What are the fundamental differences between the NHS and private healthcare?

- What three words would you use to describe the NHS?

Research

◆ Do some research online to find out what healthcare was like for people before the NHS. Write a short paragraph describing what you have learnt and share with your class.

◆ In pairs, find some examples of how science and technology advances in the NHS have improved health and saved lives. Share and compare the examples you have found with the rest of your class.

◆ Conduct a search online to find out how many people worked for the NHS when it launched in 1948 and how many people work there today.

◆ Look online to find out how many patients the NHS sees and treats every 24hrs.

◆ Talk to friends and family about their experiences of the NHS, either as patients, staff or both. Think of six questions to ask them and then write a short report on what you have discovered.

◆ In small groups, do some research into staffing shortages in the NHS. Compile a list of your findings and consider the reasons for staff shortages and how the problem might be tackled.

Design

◆ Design a poster which would encourage people to apply for jobs in the NHS.

◆ Create a social media publicity campaign persuading young people of the importance of looking after their health. Include examples of lifestyle changes they can make to improve their health and wellbeing such as eating a balanced diet and taking regular exercise.

◆ Design a children's hospital ward. Think about making it a fun, safe and comfortable place to be.

◆ Choose one of the articles in this book and create an illustration that highlights its key message.

Oral

◆ Hold a class discussion about the crisis in the NHS. Discuss staff shortages, underfunding, and how overstretched the service is because of these factors. Talk about the ways these issues could be addressed.

◆ Read the article *Top 20 public health achievements of the 21st century* on page 21. In small groups discuss any other recent improvements to public health you are aware of, and also compile a list of three or four public health achievements you would like to see happen in the next 5-10 years. Compare your ideas with rest of your class.

◆ Read the article *Healthcare systems around the world* on page 12. Discuss the following:

- Which country's healthcare service is the most similar to the UK's NHS?

- Which countries managed the COVID-19 response most successfully?

◆ 'Vaccinations should be made compulsory.' Debate this motion as a class, with one group arguing in favour and the other against.

Reading/writing

◆ Write a short paragraph definition for each of the following:

- Diabetes

- Arthritis

- Dementia

- Multiple Sclerosis

◆ Imagine you are an NHS staff member working in a busy hospital during the early days of the Coronavirus pandemic. Write a diary entry about your shift, describing the atmosphere, what you had to wear and how you felt.

Acknowledgements

The publisher is grateful for permission to reproduce the material in this book. While every care has been taken to trace and acknowledge copyright, the publisher tenders its apology for any accidental infringement or where copyright has proved untraceable. The publisher would be pleased to come to a suitable arrangement in any such case with the rightful owner.

The material reproduced in *ISSUES* books is provided as an educational resource only. The views, opinions and information contained within reprinted material in *ISSUES* books do not necessarily represent those of Independence Educational Publishers and its employees.

Images

Cover image courtesy of iStock. All other images courtesy of Freepik & Unsplash.

Illustrations

Simon Kneebone: pages 1, 14 & 26. Angelo Madrid: pages 9, 22 & 33.

Additional acknowledgements

With thanks to the Independence team: Shelley Baldry, Danielle Lobban and Jackie Staines.

Tracy Biram

Cambridge, September 2021

About National Health

The coronavirus pandemic has presented the biggest threat to our health as a nation this century. The challenges faced by the already struggling NHS have been unprecedented. This book looks at the impact of COVID-19, budget cuts and staffing shortages, as well as exploring the common health issues and illnesses that continue to ail us across the UK.

About issues

issues is a unique series of cross-curricular resource books for key stage 3, 4 & above. The series explores contemporary social issues, stimulating debate among readers of all levels. Each book presents a range of facts and opinions, providing the reader with an unbiased overview of the topic.

Titles contain articles and statistics from all key players involved in the topic covered, and include a range of diverse opinions. Elements include:

- Key facts
- Magazine features
- Charity group literature
- Cartoons and illustrations
- Journal and book extracts
- Extracts from government reports
- Statistics, including tables and graphs
- Newspaper reports and feature articles
- Accessible, easy to photocopy, full colour layouts
- Glossaries, time-lines and diagrams

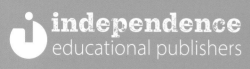

independence
educational publishers

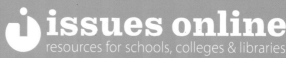

issues online
resources for schools, colleges & libraries

Orders can be placed directly with the publisher:

Independence, The Studio, High Green, Great Shelford, Cambridge, CB22 5EG, England

Fax: 01223 550806
Phone: 01223 550801
Email: issues@independence.co.uk

www.independence.co.uk
www.issuesonline.co.uk

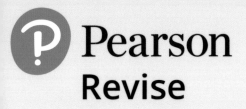

Pearson Edexcel GCSE (9–1)

History

Superpower relations and the Cold War, 1941–91

Revision Guide & Workbook + App

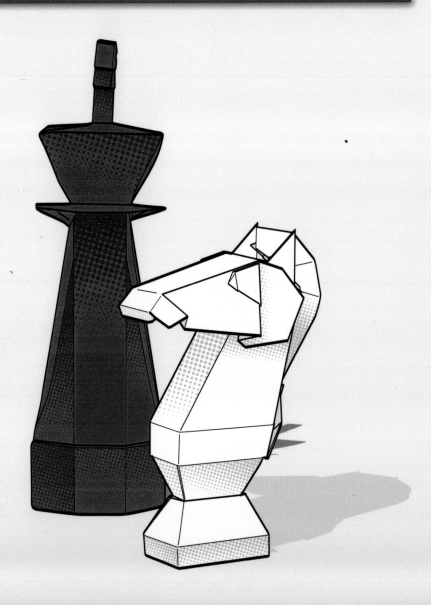

Access your revision anywhere and track your progress on the go...

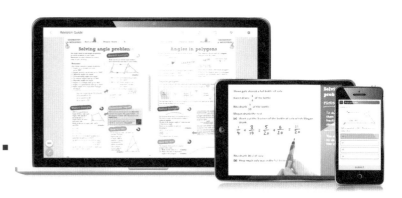

1 Download the Pearson Revise App

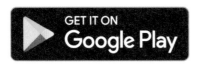

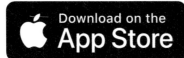

Or visit revise.pearson.com

2 Open Pearson Revise, create an account or sign in

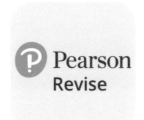

3 Redeem access code within the relevant course

4 Scratch the panel off below with a coin to reveal the code to redeem.
Do not use a knife or other sharp objects as this may damage the code.

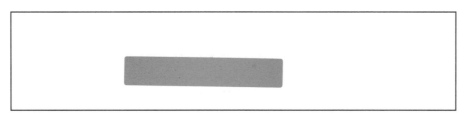

Important information

- The access code can only be used once.

- Please activate your access code as soon as possible, as it does have a use-by-date.
  If your code has expired when you enter it, please contact digital.support@pearson.com.

- The subject will be valid for three years upon activation.

- If you have bought this Revision Guide secondhand, the code may already have been used by the first owners.

Getting help

If you have any questions about accessing the Pearson Revise App or technical queries, please contact our digital support team at digital.support@pearson.com.